OXFORD MEDICAL PUBLICATIONS

Community care
for the mentally disabled

Community care for the mentally disabled

Edited by
J. K. Wing and Rolf Olsen

Oxford (New York Toronto)
OXFORD UNIVERSITY PRESS
(1979)

Oxford University Press, Walton Street, Oxford OX2 6DP

OXFORD LONDON GLASGOW
NEW YORK TORONTO MELBOURNE WELLINGTON
KUALA LUMPUR SINGAPORE JAKARTA HONG KONG TOKYO
DELHI BOMBAY CALCUTTA MADRAS KARACHI
IBADAN NAIROBI DAR ES SALAAM CAPE TOWN

British Library Cataloguing in Publication Data

Community care for the mentally disabled. – (Oxford
     medical publications).
     1. Community mental health services – Great Britain
     I. Wing, John Kenneth   II. Olson, Rolf   III. Series
     362.2'0941   RA790.7.G7   79-40392

ISBN 0-19-261189-5
ISBN 0-19-261146-1 Pbk

Phototypeset in V.I.P. Times by
Western Printing Services Ltd, Bristol
Printed and bound in Great Britain
by Billing and Sons Ltd, Guildford
and Worcester

Preface

During the past quarter of a century there has been a radical change in public and professional opinion concerning the best way to help people with chronic mental illness, mental retardation, and dementia. It has been recognized that very few need to be segregated for long periods in remote institutions and that most can look after themselves so long as a supporting network of social and medical services is available. What has not been so clearly understood is the extent to which the disabled people themselves, their relatives, and the community at large, can suffer if progress towards the new pattern of services is not made in a balanced and comprehensive way.

The contributors to this book have all conducted recent surveys into various aspects of mental disability. They summarize their views on the present state of 'community care' and make suggestions, which turn out to be surprisingly similar, concerning its future development. Although each chapter is based on research, the book is intended for those who are practically involved in running the social, medical, and voluntary services rather than for the scientists. We have kept tables and references (apart from suggestions for further reading) to a minimum. Throughout, our aim has been to describe the problems of disabled people as realistically as possible, to specify the social contexts in which these problems arise and have to be dealt with, to review the evidence for various techniques of help and prevention, and to look forward to solutions that can overcome the administrative divisions between the services at present provided.

July 1978

J. K. W.
R. O.

Contents

Contributors   viii

1 Trends in the care of the chronically mentally disabled   1
  J. K. Wing

2 Schizophrenia and the family   14
  Liz Kuipers and Diana Priestley

3 Day services and the mentally ill   36
  Carol Edwards and Jan Carter

4 Residential care for the mentally disabled   60
  Peter Ryan

5 Providing for the destitute   90
  John Leach

6 Caring for the mentally retarded   106
  Lorna Wing and Judith Gould

7 Non-hospital residential care for adults with mental
  retardation   132
  E. T. Udall and J. A. Corbett

8 Services for the elderly mentally infirm   152
  Rolf Olsen

9 Principles of the new community care   171
  J. K. Wing and Rolf Olsen

Index   187

Contributors

Jan Carter B.A., Dip. Soc. Studs., M.Sc. (Econ.)
Principal Research Officer,
National Institute for Social Work Research Unit.

J. A. Corbett F.R.C. Psych., M.R.C.P.
Consultant Psychiatrist,
Maudsley and Bethlem Royal Hospitals.

Carol Edwards B.A.
Research Officer,
National Institute for Social Work Research Unit.

Judith Gould M. Phil.
Clinical Psychologist, MRC Social Psychiatry Unit,
Institute of Psychiatry,
London.

Liz Kuipers M.Sc.
Clinical Psychologist,
MRC Social Psychiatry Unit,
Institute of Psychiatry,
London.

John Leach B.Sc. (Sociol.)
Sociologist, MRC Social Psychiatry Unit,
Institute of Psychiatry,
London.

Rolf Olsen Ph.D., M.Sc., S.R.N., Dip. Soc. Sc., Dip. Mental Health
Director Social Work Courses,
Professor of Social Work,
Social Administration Department,
University of Birmingham.

Diana Priestley B.Sc., S.R.N.
Community Worker, National Schizophrenia Fellowship,
78 Victoria Road,
Surbiton, Surrey KT6 4JT.

Peter Ryan B.A.
   Formerly Research Psychologist, MRC Social Psychiatry Unit,
   Institute of Psychiatry,
   London.

E. T. Udall M.A., CSW.
   Formerly Senior Social Worker,
   Institute of Psychiatry, London.

J. K. Wing MD, Ph.D, FRC Psych.
   Director,
   MRC Social Psychiatry Unit,
   Professor of Social Psychiatry,
   Institute of Psychiatry,
   London.

Lorna Wing MD, MRC Psych.
   Scientific Staff,
   MRC Social Psychiatry Unit,
   Institute of Psychiatry,
   London.

1 Trends in the care of the chronically mentally disabled

J. K. Wing

Thomas McKeown has pointed out that the improvements in public health in the western world during the past century and a half have not been due mainly to advances in diagnosis and treatment (important though these are) but to an improvement in standards of nutrition, a healthier physical environment such as a clean water supply, and a decline in family size. McKeown is concerned particularly with the decline in mortality rates, which cannot be expected to continue at the same rate although there is still room for some improvement. The three great health problems that remain are all in the field of chronic handicap: congenital disability including severe mental retardation; chronic mental illness; and the illnesses of late middle-age and the senium, including dementia.

Two of the central principles of the originators of the Welfare State in this country (the authors of the minority report of the Poor Law Commission of 1909) were that prevention is cheaper and more effective than cure and that charitable activity has its proper place in supporting a public service. The historical development of the British national health and social services can best be understood in the light of these two principles.

The first public hospitals for the mentally ill and retarded were set up in the early part of the nineteenth century in reaction against what were thought to be the intolerable conditions under which the mentally ill and retarded were then treated 'in the community'. In the new small hospitals, what was known as 'moral treatment' became the ideal. An educational approach was adopted, physical restraint was disavowed, and an attitude of optimism about the outcome prevailed. The discharge rates were as high as those reached today.

Why this early promise not only did not fulfil itself but was actually reversed towards the end of the nineteenth century is still not completely clear, though a change in public attitudes which resulted in the restrictive Lunacy Acts of 1890 and 1891 has been blamed. Perhaps a degree of overoptimism on the part of the early reformers also contributed, because it led to disillusion and a swing towards overpessimism. Certainly, it soon became difficult to maintain the small size of the early hospitals. David Rothman has suggested that many different types of institution underwent a similar change. Early nineteenth-century theories of training and segregation were initially based on the idea that much social deviance (including insanity and crime) was due to pressures resulting from the new freedoms fostered by the Enlightenment. But the corrective regimes became identified as desirable in themselves, long after the increasing flow of admissions and decreasing proportion of discharges had demonstrated that they were unable to prevent or cure deviation. 'The organizing concepts of the asylum disguised and even subtly encouraged a custodial operation. The exaggerated emphasis on physical structure, on the benefits inherent in institutions, promoted an attitude that automatically identified an asylum with a therapeutic milieu. Many superintendents suffered a declining number of attendants together with a swelling number of inmates without altering their belief that the setting itself was ameliorative.'

The subsequent custodial era, characterized by large mental hospitals with a relatively low turnover of patients, lasted for half a century until the Mental Treatment Act of 1930 foreshadowed a new liberalism. The influx of a new generation of psychiatrists after the Second World War, together with the establishment of a National Health Service, led to a new attitude towards the mental health services and a determination to bring them into line with the newly developing welfare state. The ideas of Thomas Main and Maxwell Jones, who emphasized social methods in the treatment of the neurotic and personality disorders (e.g. in helping returning prisoners of war) spread to the mental hospitals. G. M. Bell, Donal Early, R. K. Freudenberg, Duncan Macmillan, and T. P. Rees, among others, again emphasized the ideas of the early pioneers: open doors, the therapeutic community, rehabilitation through the provision of meaningful domestic, social, and occupational roles, early resettlement outside hospital through the use of day centres, half-way houses and sheltered work, and full social support for relatives. Virtually all the ideas now current in 'community care' were introduced in the 1950s by pioneering psychiatrists.

At Mapperley Hospital in Nottingham, the number of beds began to decline long before reserpine and phenothiazines were introduced in 1955. The new medications accelerated these social advances and made it possible for other hospitals to follow the lead of the pioneers. The Mental Health Act of 1959 set a seal of approval on practices that had already been adopted in the most progressive hospitals.

Following the recognition of a statistical trend towards decreasing numbers of in-patients, the Hospital Plan of 1962 looked forward to a time when psychiatric units attached to district general hospitals would be able to meet most of the specialist medical needs of the local population, together with community hospitals for those with severe dementia. The social functions of the large hospitals would be taken over by the Social Services Departments of local authorities created in 1970. Finally, the three branches of the National Health Service—general practice, hospital services, and public health—were integrated, theoretically at least, into one administrative structure in 1974.

In this way, it was hoped that the large mental hospitals would eventually be replaced by a network of other services. In 1961, the Minister of Health was confident that the statistical trends, together with new government plans, would lead to 'nothing less than the elimination of by far the greater number of this country's mental hospitals as they stand today'. At the end of 1975, however, there were still 188 patients per 100 000 general population in psychiatric hospitals: 59 of them (31 per cent) had been resident for less than one year—the 'short-stay' group; 39 (21 per cent) for more than one but less than five years—the 'new' long-stay group; and 90 (48 per cent) for more than five years—the 'old' long-stay group. Not a single mental hospital had been closed.

In the same year, 1975, a government White Paper admitted that 'by and large the nonhospital community resources are still minimal . . . The failure . . . to develop anything approaching adequate services is perhaps the greatest disappointment of the last 15 years'. The White Paper recommended 4–6 beds per 100 000 population in short-stay hostels and 15–24 beds per 100 000 in longer-stay non-hospital accommodation, but in March 1975 only one region could count on as many as half the number of recommended places. Overall, local authorities were providing, at that time, 28 per cent of the minimum, and 18 per cent of the maximum, requirement. Even when provision by voluntary bodies was added, fewer than half of the minimum number of residential places were available. Day care facilities were equally scarce; 63 local authorities made no such provision at all. The situation of the mentally retarded and the elderly mentally infirm was no more advantageous than that of the chronically mentally ill.

We are particularly concerned in this book with the social needs of people with long-term 'mental disablement'. This term covers those who are disabled by reason of mental retardation, dementia (mental infirmity), and chronic mental illness. We shall not use the term 'mental handicap', because it is used officially to refer only to the mentally retarded, although it should have a more general meaning. To refer to those disabled by chronic schizophrenia as 'mentally ill' induces an expectation that medical treatment is the chief factor determining the type of residential or day care needed, whereas it is generally agreed that social needs are often more important. 'Mental disability' is a more neutral and general term, carrying much the same connotation as 'physical disability' and with the same implication of a very wide range of social and medical needs.

The term 'care' will also be used in a general sense, to include all the forms of help given to disabled people; treatment, counsel, support, rehabilitation, shelter, and welfare benefits.

The principal concern of this book is with non-hospital forms of care but it is impossible to understand the present situation and future needs without first understanding the changes that have taken place in hospital practice. The rest of this chapter will be devoted to a brief account of the ideas and methods that have dominated hospital practice during the past twenty-five years. Developments in hospitals for the 'adult mentally ill' will be used by way of example but similar points can be made about each of the other two broad categories of mental disablement—mental retardation and mental infirmity in the elderly.

The 'old' long-stay

The differentiation between 'old' and 'new' long-stay is, of course, arbitrary and, since it depends on innovations that were introduced at a different pace in different parts of the country, no one dividing line is generally applicable. Nevertheless, there is a valid distinction to be drawn between those who accumulated at a time when the major emphasis was not placed on resettlement outside hospital and those who have accumulated more recently, in spite of all efforts to the contrary.

Erving Goffman was one of the most influential theorists of the 1960s, partly because of the excellence of his prose, which few sociologists writing about psychiatry have since been able to match, but principally because the core of his argument was based on practices in 'total institutions', which everyone knew, as soon as they were pointed out, to be indefensible. He showed that much time and trouble could be saved 'if everyone's soiled clothing can be indiscriminately placed in one bundle and laundered clothing can be redistributed, not according to ownership but according to rough size'. Goffman did not attempt to test hypotheses, his style was literary rather than scientific, and he did not report on hospitals where the practices he criticized had been replaced by more humane and effective methods. But he had the enormous merit of considering that patients are entitled to a reasonable human dignity. They should not be treated as numbers.

Empirical studies of the long-stay population began to be carried out during the late 1950s. They demonstrated that patients were disabled in several different ways. First there were impairments that seemed to be part of the illness itself. One of these (an 'invisible' impairment), was liability to relapse with acute symptoms of schizophrenia, or paranoid psychosis, or mania, or depression, following discharge from hospital. This was often regarded as sufficient reason for a long stay. More obvious were chronic 'negative' impairments such as those that commonly accompany and follow acute schizophrenia: psychomotor slowness, underactivity, poor ability to communicate using verbal or non-verbal language, and social withdrawal. In very severe cases, patients were mute, incontinent, and apparently incapable of independent volition, even having to be spoon-fed. Severe and recurrent depression or excitement also occurred.

It was found that social understimulation, characteristic of the poorer hospitals, made the negative impairments worse, while realistic social stimulation (i.e. up to a standard that was actually achievable) reduced them quite quickly to a minimal or base-line level, the severity of which varied from patient to patient. Some improved a great deal when new regimes of 'resocialization' were introduced into a poor hospital; most improved to some extent; a few did not respond at all. It was perhaps inevitable that progress such as this, which could be quite dramatic when a patient who had seemed for years to be severely disabled 'came alive' again, should lead some people to assume that all impairment had been created by institutional pressures; even that abolishing hospitals would prevent impairment altogether.

It was sometimes forgotten that the substantial effects of 'rehabilitation' found in several experiments were due to the removal of an extra, unnecessary component of impairment that had been added (on top of an irreducible minimum) by living in an understimulating social environment. By the same token, it was often not recognized that understimulation is not a necessary feature of wards in large institutions (although staff ratios sometimes make it unavoidable) and that it can occur in any day or residential setting and even in the family home. The term 'institution' became synonymous with 'hospital' (i.e. all hospitals were regarded as 'total institutions'), while non-hospital accommodation was assumed automatically and unthinkingly, to be 'part of the community'.

Another major result of the early surveys and experiments was also overlooked. This was to identify two other components in disablement. One was 'extrinsic' social disadvantage and deprivation, which had often been present for many years before the individual was first admitted to hospital and which had its own complex causes, many of them social in nature. People who had never established firm social roots were far less likely to be visited after admission, less likely to retain contacts with the outside world through letters or visits out, and more vulnerable to pressure towards conformity to institutional life. Vocational, social, and domestic 'rehabilitation' was often effective in making up for past deprivation as well as in developing unsuspected talents. Sometimes, however, long-term disadvantages could not be corrected by the hospital's rehabilitation programme.

The final component in disablement arose from adverse personal reactions to impairment and disadvantage and was therefore secondary. For example, the longer a patient had been in hospital, the more likely he was to want to stay and to have no plans for the future. This was true even of those who were not any longer severely impaired. Such people had not, for years, practised going on buses, shopping, or exercising the role of husband, wife, parent, employee, or customer. They took little interest in the affairs of the outside world, even to the extent of not updating everyday knowledge such as the price of a postage stamp or a bus ride to the shops. This gradual acquisition of contentment with hospital life and loss of the wish to live any other was named 'institutionalism'. Only prolonged and gradual resocialization could counter it. Once again, however, it was not always recognized that such secondary reactions were not specific to hospitals but could occur in many other settings as well. They reflected, above all, the expectations of important people in the immediate social environment.

Thus the three components of disability had different causes and required different techniques of rehabilitation. The social disablement resulting from various combinations of causes might look much the same but it was necessary to discover which of the component factors was most amenable to help. In some cases, intrinsic impairment was so severe and chronic that long years of devoted effort seemed to make little impact and the best that could be achieved was life in a sheltered setting, aimed simply at preventing further deterioration. At the other extreme, when the disability was mainly secondary, rehabilitation could be dramatically successful.

The characteristics of hospitals which were recognized as particularly harmful were social understimulation (which fostered inactivity and social withdrawal), restrictive practices (which decreased the opportunities for multiple role-playing and the exercise of independence), depersonalization (which gave no encouragement to the development of personal initiative or identity), and authoritarianism and pauperism (which emphasized the individual's status at the bottom of the social scale, allowed no expression of personal taste. and rubbed home the fact that all privileges were dependent on the charity of others). Physical neglect and even ill-treatment were less common factors but very serious when they did occur.

The best hospitals did learn how to control these factors, insofar as it was possible with the resources and staff ratios available. Size did not seem to be an important factor independently of the others. Some of the most innovative hospitals were quite large, but wards were split up and maximum use was made of villas and units outside the main grounds. Nevertheless, size, barrack-like buildings, and geographical remoteness have an invisible effect on the attitudes of staff and patients even in good hospitals.

The achievements of the staff of psychiatric hospitals, at the time when a wind of change was blowing, were solid and substantial. Most of the ideas now used in 'community care' are derived from the innovations, experiments, and evaluations of those years. Sheltered residential care—in the hostels of the Mental After-Care Association and other agencies, in family care, in boarding accommodation, in group homes, and in hotels—received a new impetus. (Many of these options had, of course, been tried over a century ago.) Half-way houses were introduced in order to carry on rehabilitative processes begun in hospital. Similarly, the specification of the principles of vocational rehabilitation, the use of Industrial Rehabilitation Units (now Employment Rehabilitation Centres), the placement of patients in 'Remploy' factories and industrial 'enclaves', the setting up of sheltered workshops manufacturing their own products, the establishment of day centres and social clubs, were all innovations stimulated by the urgent need to find ways of helping 'old' long-stay patients to re-establish themselves outside hospital.

As more hospitals have adopted the techniques of the pioneers, it has become less easy to resettle the smaller and smaller group of ageing long-stay people who have not responded or who wish to remain where they are. The size of the hospital population in England has almost been halved since 1954 and the task of maintaining the momentum becomes increasingly difficult. Remarkable and unexpected improvements still reward years of effort but the returns are diminishing.

Changes in hospital services for 'old' long-stay residents in mental retardation hospitals have followed a similar pattern. Shortly after the Second World War, Neil O'Connor and Jack Tizard found that it was quite common for people whose intellectual ability was only moderately impaired to remain resident for years. This is no longer the case although many people who have accumulated from the old days do still remain. Because of the limited expectation of life, people with dementia are found mainly in the 'new' long-stay group.

The 'new' long-stay

Meanwhile, in the psychiatric hospitals, a much smaller 'new' long-stay group has been accumulating. Of the 39 people per 100 000 population who, at the end of 1975, had been in hospital for more than one but less than five years, twenty-five were less than 65 years old. Several surveys have been focused upon the needs of this younger group in order to try to answer the question: 'Why do they stay so long when every effort is made by hospital staff to prevent them doing so?'

A psychiatrist and a social worker, Sheila Mann and Wendy Cree, undertook a survey of 'new' long-stay patients under 65 in one hospital selected at random from each of the regions in England and Wales. They found that nearly half (44 per cent) were diagnosed as schizophrenic, the next largest category (16 per cent) being people with depressive and manic conditions. A substantial minority (14 per cent) were suffering from an early form of dementia and 7 per cent were said to have 'personality disorders'. The remainder had multiple diagnoses of which psychiatric disorder was only one and not necessarily the most important (e.g. alcoholism, epilepsy, blindness, deafness, physical disability, mental retardation, etc.)

In general, these people were socially isolated, unmarried, out of touch or at odds with their families or friends, and had few occupational skills. These social disadvantages must have had something to do with their becoming long-stay. So must their personal reaction to discharge: only 29 per cent had a clear wish to leave. This 'institutionalism' had developed much more rapidly than in the old long-stay group and was not, therefore, simply due to being cut-off from the outside world (very few of the hospitals surveyed conformed to Goffman's concept of a total institution), but to a reaction to impairments and disadvantages.

After interviewing each patient and talking to the doctors, nurses, and social workers concerned, the two investigators made their own judgement as to needs for residential or day care, assuming that unlimited resources were available. They concluded that there were four major groups. First, one-third of the patients sampled seemed to need further hospital treatment or care, with the possibility of eventual discharge. This included people on compulsory orders (half the group), those with severely disturbed behaviour, and those with florid psychotic symptoms.

It was thought that a second group (22 per cent of the sample) needed a degree of supervision, because of a tendency to self-neglect, wandering, inactivity, or failure to continue medication, or a need for supportive personal relations with a member of staff. It would be important, in this group, to detect early signs of relapse. Some members had delusional beliefs which they did not express except to trusted staff members. Very few would have been able to hold down a job and most would therefore need to go to an occupation or rehabilitation centre. Some would need transport from hostel to day centre. Such people are not, at the moment, acceptable in local authority hostels (see Chapter 4). Moreover, the placement is likely to be long-term, if not permament.

The third group of new long-stay patients (15 per cent) had improved since admission and were ready for discharge to less super-vised accommodation such as group homes, boarding homes, or their own families. This was not such a handicapped group as the first two and there was a less marked history of social disadvantage. Two-thirds could probably have managed at least sheltered work.

Finally, there was the group of people with multiple disabilities (25 per cent). Over half had pre-senile dementia and needed similar accommodation to the elderly mentally infirm. The rest had a diversity of needs which could have been met by specialist facilities (e.g. for the blind, the 'younger chronic sick', the severely retarded, etc.) had they been available.

These four groups, between them, accounted for 95 per cent of the new long-stay population under the age of 65. (The other 5 per cent were on extended leave.) Apart from the small third group, the out-standing features were severe impairment together with social disad-vantage. The heterogeneous fourth group ought to be cared for by more specific types of service. The label of 'psychotic' had become attached to people whose main problem was quite different. Most (apart from those with early dementia) had little psychiatric disorder and did not need to be in hospital any longer.

The first two groups presented more difficult problems, both theoretically and practically. There probably is a new long-stay group needing prolonged hospital treatment or security. It is small enough to be dealt with locally rather than regionally but, because of the length of stay, requires domestic-scale accommodation, perhaps in a hospital annexe. A hospital ward is not appropriate. Consideration for transfer to this type of accommodation needs to be given much earlier; for example, six months after admission, by which time it should be clear, in most cases, what the prognosis is likely to be.

The second group does not necessarily need to be in hospital at all but local authorities and voluntary bodies are reluctant to accept people with such severe problems, particularly if they have to attend day centres as well, with all the associated transport difficulties. Since the patients are the responsibility of hospital staff, it would seem reasonable for hospitals to be given the responsibility for setting up the appropriate (domestic-scale) accommodation. Where the hospital site is within the catchment area, a house located on the boundary, with its front door opening on the public street and its back door opening on the hospital's private grounds, would seem ideal. Spacious grounds are important, since they give the patients room to move about in the open without being directly in the public eye. Another advantage of being on the hospital site is that extra staff are available at times of crisis and a wide range of activities is available during the daytime and in leisure hours. When the hospital is far from its catchment area, setting up such a 'hospital-hostel' would be complicated and costly, because of high staff ratios when emergency staff are not available, the need for large grounds, and the expense of providing transport to day centres.

A 'new long-stay' hostel was set up at the Maudsley Hospital in the autumn of 1977 and is being evaluated in order to discover whether the idea is feasible. Because there is a register of all people from the catchment area who contact psychiatric services it will be possible to put the experiment into context and thus to determine how many of the new long-stay can benefit.

People admitted to mental retardation hospitals nowadays are not only severely or profoundly handicapped intellectually but have physical disabilities or disturbed behaviour as well. The 'new' long-stay group is therefore composed of those who are non-ambulant, or aggressive, destructive, or otherwise difficult to live with. As in the case of the mentally 'ill', hostel accommodation is rarely available for disorders of this severity. Further consideration will be found in §8 of Chapter 6.

Because of the high mortality rate, most people with severe dementia who need to be in hospital are resident for less than five years. There are a few places in the British Isles where admission for dementia can be arranged easily and with little or no delay but in general the problem is now one of lack of adequate hospital accommodation. The problems are discussed in Chapter 8.

Implications for other forms of care

Short-term and long-term hospital treatment and care are means of reducing disablement and its social consequences. They can be used to maximum effect only if they are regarded as *part* of 'community care' rather than being somehow opposed to it and only if other resources are closely integrated within one overall pattern of services. Much of our knowledge of impairment has been developed through medical research into mental illness, mental retardation, and dementia (see, for example, Chapters 2, 6, and 8). A rational provision for these conditions must be based on knowledge of the way that social as well as clinical factors can act to precipitate and maintain disablement. This means that social disadvantages and secondary reactions need to be taken into account as well as clinical impairments.

In the past, the mental hospital and mental retardation hospital have had to try to deal with a very wide range of social as well as medical functions, and they still act as a stop-gap when other sections of the service are not available. Unfortunately, the hospitals have been running down while the parallel build up in the overlapping facilities has lagged far behind. This is partly due to the fact that much of the innovative drive behind the new ideas has come from the hospital service (which is financed centrally) while local authorities have only reluctantly taken on their new responsibilities. It is partly due, as the White Paper on 'Better Services for the Mentally Ill' suggests, to the slow acceptance by public opinion of community responsibility for maintaining the social ties and quality of life of disabled people. But it is also partly due to an unrealistic assumption that all mental disability can be prevented if the hospitals are abolished.

The evidence that groups of disabled people outside hospital are at risk of relapse or of increasing chronic disablement because day and residential facilities (which used to be provided on one hospital site) are not being provided elsewhere is overwhelming. Julian Leff and Christine Vaughn interviewed people who had previously been admitted to hospital for schizophrenic or manic-depressive psychoses but who had not been in contact with psychiatrists for a year or more. About one-third were judged to need help with housing or social problems. In another study, of disabled people who had been out of work for years although not in hospital, the need for sheltered residential accommodation was very clear. Studies of relatives' problems indicated a particular need among disabled people living with elderly relatives who feared what would happen when they were no longer able to provide care and supervision. A substantial proportion of destitute men (the number of whom is increasing as unemployment rises and becomes a long-term feature of society) are suffering from mental disabilities. Burdens on families are particularly evident when the patient is over 65.

This book is devoted to a consideration of the principles of care for the chronically disabled, which are not different in nature (though the specifics do, of course, vary), whatever the day or residential setting in which they are applied. The ideas behind the National Health Service are applicable also to the National Social Service. There should be geographical responsibility (every individual in need should be able to obtain help from a designated service), comprehensive coverage (a variety of services covering every type of need), and integrated care (so that movement through the network of social and medical services is facilitated and there are no gaps or sudden changes in level of expectation to interrupt what would otherwise be a smooth progress towards an optimum settlement). We shall consider in Chapter 9 the extent to which these elements can be combined into an effective means of minimizing disability, maximizing independence, and reducing unnecessary burdens on relatives and the community at large.

FURTHER READING

Bennett, D. H. and Wing, J. K. (1963). Sheltered workshops for the psychiatrically handicapped. In *Trends in the mental health services* (eds. H. Freeman and J. Farndale). Pergamon Press, London.

Brown, G. W., Bone, M., Dalison, B., and Wing, J. K. (1966). *Schizophrenia and social care*. Oxford University Press, London.

Creer, C. and Wing, J. K. (1974). *Schizophrenia at home*. National Schizophrenia Fellowship, 78 Victoria Road, Surbiton, Surrey KT6 4JT.

DHSS (1975). *Better services for the mentally ill*. Cmnd 6233. HMSO, London.

Leff, J. P. and Vaughn, C. (1972). Psychiatric patients in-contact and out-of-contact with services: a clinical and social assessment. In *Evaluating a community psychiatric service* (eds. J. K. Wing and A. M. Hailey). Oxford University Press, London.

Mann, S. and Cree, W. (1976). 'New' long-stay patients: a national sample of 15 mental hospitals in England and Wales, 1972–3. *Psychol. Med.* **6**, 603–16.

McKeown, T. (1976). *The role of medicine: dream, mirage or nemesis?* Nuffield Provincial Hospitals Trust, London.

O'Connor, N. and Tizard, J. (1956). *The social problem of mental deficiency*. Pergamon Press, London.

Rothman, D. J. (1971). *The discovery of the asylum: social order and disorder in the New Republic*. Little, Brown & Company, Mass.

Wing, J. K. (1974). Sheltered environments for the psychiatrically handicapped. In *Providing a comprehensive district psychiatric service*. DHSS.: HMSO, London.

— (1978). *Reasoning about madness*. Oxford University Press, Oxford.

— (1978). *Schizophrenia: towards a new synthesis*. Academic Press, London.

— and Brown, G. W. (1970). *Institutionalism and schizophrenia*. Cambridge University Press, London.

— Bennett, D. H., and Denham, J. (1964). *The industrial rehabilitation of long-stay schizophrenicccc patients*. M. R. C. Memo. No. 42. HMSO, London.

Wing, L., Wing, J. K., Griffiths, D. and Stevens, B. (1972). An epidemiological and experimental evaluation of industrial rehabilitation of chronic psychotic patients in the community. In *Evaluating a community psychiatric service* (eds. J. K. Wing and A. M. Hailey). Oxford University Press, London.

2 Schizophrenia and the family

PART I *Liz Kuipers*
PART II *Diana Priestley*

The first part of this chapter deals with the problems presented by people with schizophrenia who are living at home, usually with parents or a spouse. The second part is based on a pioneer project in which a professional community worker worked with a group of relatives who met together in an effort to come to terms with the problems of 'living with schizophrenia'.

PART I The problems of relatives

Schizophrenia is the most seriously handicapping psychiatric condition beginning in adult life. Half of the patients living in psychiatric hospitals are both long-stay (in the sense that they have been resident for more than a year) and diagnosed as schizophrenic. Many of them have accumulated in former times, when attitudes were more pessimistic and treatment less successful than now. But there is a substantial 'new' long-stay group accumulating as well. If we take a length of stay in hospital of more than one year but less than five years as a criterion, at the end of 1975 there were 18185 people in this group (39 for every 100000 population). Further, 'new' long-stay groups are accumulating in alternative residential accommodation, such as hostels and group homes, and also in day centres, as we shall see in the next two chapters. Yet others become destitute. They become long-stay 'on the streets' (see Chapter 5). The need of these people for various forms of shelter is very often due to the chronic symptoms or chronic impairments of schizophrenia.

However, most people with chronic schizophrenia live at home. They and their relatives acquire a wealth of experience about how to live with such a condition. It would be wasteful not to try to learn from those who have been most successful in order to help, not only other relatives and patients, but also professional people who are responsible for residential and day care settings.

The most dramatic and intensely distressing symptoms of schizophrenia occur during a sudden attack when the affected individual experiences his thoughts being interfered with or distorted, or alien thoughts being put into his mind, or his thoughts being broadcast for all to hear. Other experiences are that his will is not his own; that some other agency or force compels him to think, or act, or feel in ways that are completely alien. Auditory hallucinations (the experience of hearing voices that others cannot hear and for which there is no demonstrable source) are common. The temptation to put forward delusional explanations for these experiences, in terms of supernatural powers such as spirits, physical forces such as television, radio-waves, or microphones, or occult influences such as telepathy, is very great. Cultural attitudes partially determine the explanation adopted. The basic experiences, however, are real, and they are much the same all over the world. Someone affected by such experiences may act on the basis of delusions or hallucinations and will then appear to behave in a bizarre and irrational way, although he may regard his behaviour as quite reasonable.

Such experiences are often self-limiting, particularly if the affected person can be given a period of peace in which to recover. The phenothiazine drugs are a useful means of bringing them under control. However, other less dramatic symptoms often precede such acute attacks, accompany them, and sometimes persist afterwards as well. The first of these is a difficulty in thinking coherently and systematically. The train of thought is disconnected and it is impossible to reach a logical conclusion. The second is very common; the individual becomes very slow in thought and movement, lacks the energy to complete ordinary tasks, is underactive and socially withdrawn, These chronic symptoms (or impairments) are severely handicapping because they interfere with the individual's ability to maintain social relationships, to work, and to engage in interesting recreations.

These impairments—whether delusions or hallucinations, 'thought disorder', or slowness and social withdrawal—are not obvious to other people, as they would be in someone who had lost a limb or his eyesight, or who has some wasting physical disease. The affected individuals may therefore be expected to behave 'normally' and be exposed to great pressure by employers, or relatives, or caring staff, to achieve normal standards of social performance that are quite impossible for them. Attitudes of this kind are, of course, cultural and affected by education. A condition such as diabetes can also be very handicapping, and require long-term medication, but most people understand that diabetics have to take special diets and avoid certain situations, and they willingly and sympathetically make allowances.

The same is not yet true of conditions like schizophrenia and prejudice may be found among the general population, relatives, and professional people, alike.

Some of the problems of relatives were described in a survey of 80 families containing a schizophrenic member (Creer and Wing 1974). Over 70 per cent said that social withdrawal was the problem most frequently encountered, followed by underactivity and lack of conversation. Threats of violence were a problem for about a quarter of relatives. Sexually unusual behaviour or suicidal attempts were encountered quite rarely, although about one-third of the relatives said that depression was a problem. Some people spent all day in their rooms, 'either crouching on the bed or endlessly playing records to drown the "voices"'. Others refused to meet visitors or even to talk to their own relatives. Some engaged in repetitive activities such as making cups of tea; others would sit for long hours doing nothing at all but stare into space. Although many had lost the ability to make new friends and feared social contact, they nevertheless felt lonely. Relatives knew this, but often being the only ones in contact with them found it very demanding—'on the occasions when I do go out in the evening I am conscious of my daughter's lonely presence at home'. A lot of relatives just stopped going out altogether.

In reaction to these problems, most relatives had experienced anxiety, depression, guilt, and anger by turns. Frequently reported was a feeling of apprehension, or 'living on my nerves' caused by the unexpectedness of behaviour. As one relative wrote: 'She veers from total silence at times to talking nonstop for literally hours and days and nights at a time', or 'simple things like getting up in the morning, washing, getting dressed, going to bed without disturbing others in the house—one cannot assume any of these will happen'. Another mother wrote: 'without warning she would change mood'. This sort of problem is made worse by the fact that the affected individuals often do not know that there is anything the matter, or fluctuate in awareness, and it is left to whoever is with them to establish what their feelings are.

At present then it appears that the typical situation when someone with chronic schizophrenia is living at home, either all the time or between hospital admissions, is of a man or woman aged about 30 living with one or both parents aged 60 or more years. The individual has to cope with the after-effects of his illness, the possibility of relapse, continuous medication, and difficulties in picking up the threads of a normal life again. The parents have to cope with a grown-up son or daughter who is socially isolated and dependent on their care, but often demanding of time and energy and unpredictable from day to day regarding behaviour or mood. This is probably the worst picture since many people do recover completely. However, it is the most severely handicapped who need most services, and they are the focus of this chapter. We do now have some information about living with schizophrenia, and about the best ways of coping with problems as they arise. If this information were more widely used it would be possible to alleviate some of the more difficult problems.

Family influence on mental illness

Over the years there has been considerable interest, not only in the problems that families containing a schizophrenic member face, but also in the influence that families have on the condition itself. Since no physical causes have yet been discovered, it has been suggested that other factors, such as the family environment itself, were responsible. Laing and Esterson, for example, saw schizophrenia in terms of a valid response to family and societal pressures, rather than as an illness to be treated by medication or other treatments. The difficulty with theories of this kind is that they are retrospective; they depend upon studies of families now containing a schizophrenic member and trying to reconstruct the past. Memories of what occurred 20 to 30 years earlier are very unreliable and the investigator may sometimes rely too much on his own theories in deciding what happened. The risk of confusing behaviour which may have caused the illness with behaviour that may have resulted from it is also evident. If the son has schizophrenia and his mother is very protective, is this because he is schizophrenic, or is he schizophrenic because she is protective? One way of overcoming the problem is to undertake a long-term study; following up a large group of people randomly selected from the population, in order to discover what family characteristics are common when children later develop schizophrenia. The difficulty is that only one in 100 people in the general population develop schizophrenia, so that very large numbers of people have to be followed up in this way and the results are a long time coming. Some long-term studies are, in fact, being carried out, but the results will not be known for many years.

The work that has been done in order to determine whether families cause schizophrenia was recently reviewed by Hirsch and Leff, who came to the following conclusions:

1. More parents of schizophrenic patients are psychiatrically disturbed than parents of normal children and more of the mothers show 'schizoid' personality traits.

2. The parents of schizophrenic patients show more concern and disharmony than the parents of other psychiatric patients.

3. The pre-schizophrenic child suffers more frequently from physical ill health or mild disability early in life than the normal child.

4. Mothers of schizophrenic children show more concern and protectiveness than mothers of normal children, both in the current situation and in their attitudes to the children before they fell ill.

Two possible explanations for a relationship between traits in the parents and subsequent schizophrenia in the offspring are that genetic factors are involved and that parents are reacting to their child's abnormality. In fact, both explanations are likely to contribute. Certainly, it can be shown that parents of children with physical disabilities are also protective, sometimes with good reason; sometimes too much so.

An alternative way of looking at the family influences on schizophrenia however is to concentrate on the effect of the family on the *course* of the symptoms and impairments: what the family can do to make the condition improve or get worse once the first attack has occurred. This has been studied in considerable detail during the last twenty years and much evidence has now been accumulated.

In the 1950s, it was noticed that when long-stay male schizophrenic patients were discharged from hospital, whether they managed to stay out of hospital successfully or whether they relapsed and had to be readmitted seemed to be related to the type of living group they returned to. Specifically, those who did worst were those who returned to the close emotional ties of a spouse or of parents, rather than living alone or in a hostel. In a further study, patients and relatives were interviewed just before discharge, and then together in the home two weeks later. It was found that some relatives expressed a lot of emotion when talking about the schizophrenic members of the family. The patient living in a high-emotion family was much more likely to relapse within a year of discharge or to be readmitted because of a return of bizarre behaviour.

Further studies were then undertaken in order to check these findings. The interview with the relative was refined and other factors which might have contributed to the relapse were checked. The result was still the same. It seemed that if a relative was rated as expressing a high amount of emotion in a home interview, shortly before a patient was discharged, and if the patient then returned to this intense atmosphere, relapse was far more likely. This occurred in about half the families. Conversely it appeared that in the other half of the families, rated as low on expressed emotion, the patient was far less likely to relapse.

The ratings of expressed emotion in these families was based on the kinds of judgements that we all make about each other to some extent, only for these purposes they were defined in a much more explicit and precise way: the tone of the respondent's voice, the speed of speech, the amount of distress shown, and the way in which things are said during the interview. It is clear that even a simple sentence, such as 'I'm going out now', can have many different meanings depending on the tone of voice and the emphasis on different words. These aspects are much more important than the content of what is said (which is rated as well but for other purposes). When the interview was first developed, many different emotions were rated, including warmth, dissatisfaction, hostility, criticism, and emotional over-involvement. However, eventually two factors were found to be of prime importance: first, the amount of criticism and second, the amount of emotional over-involvement by the relatives. Criticism is rated when a relative makes a derogatory or disapproving remark about the patient with some negative feeling shown in the tone and emphasis of the voice, e.g. 'I can't *stand* the way he does that'. Over-involvement is rated if extremely protective or over-concerned behaviour is shown by the relative but only if this is greater what would ordinarily be shown when someone is admitted to hospital. Obviously, most people would be upset and anxious at an acute hospital admission, and only extreme examples of intrusiveness or involvement are rated. For example, a father said about his daughter: 'We were always together. She didn't like other people. I don't think there's much wrong with her at all. I miss her. I think about her all the time.' Or a mother about her son: 'I watch him all the time. I worry and I watch him in case he does it again . . . I've been worried sick about him.'

The fact that patients living with highly critical or over-involved relatives are likely to have higher relapse rates does not necessarily mean that the relatives have different personalities to those who are more emotionally neutral. Living with a mentally ill person can be extremely stressful and upsetting, and some of the things that occur would be found irritating or intolerable by nearly everyone. What seems to be happening is that given this difficult behaviour in a mentally ill relative, some relatives react in one way and others very differently. Some families learn over the years how to cope, usually by trial and error, and it depends on what point in the course the measurements are made. However, a few relatives never seem to learn. This may partly be due to the fact that they have not received any help (see

Part II of this chapter). Some degree of irritable reaction is completely understandable, particularly when relatives become angry and upset at the irrational behaviour they have had to contend with. What is surprising is that some of them either automatically or over the years do find out how to manage and can co-exist reasonably well with the ups and downs of mental illness. Further, since we know that many families, characterized as low in expressed emotion, have developed useful ways of coping, it should be possible to use that knowledge for the benefit of the other families who have more difficulty.

About one-quarter of the relatives expressed no criticism at all despite having lived with some very severe behaviour problems. Looking at these particular families more closely, the hypothesis of a rather negative, flat, and uninvolved family life is not supported. The opposite of high-expressed emotion is not just lack of criticism and involvement, but more a positive concern and care for the individual, expressed without intrusiveness. One father said: 'I feel so sorry for him about the whole affair.' A mother expressed this concern by her actions: 'I try to buck her up . . . I coax her a bit, give her a cup of tea.'

Such relatives have learned when to leave the patient alone 'until the mood passes'. One mother said: 'I'm as close to him as anyone, but we may be in the same room for hours without talking' and: 'I just let him go his own way, I don't interfere.' To some extent there was a lowered expectation; patients were not thought to be as capable as they were before, but the remedy was not to argue and get annoyed but to encourage as high a standard as was feasible and not go beyond this limit.

An elderly widow living with her sister said of her: 'I don't worry her with anything really. I just give her jobs to do that I think she can do and if she doesn't want to do them, she doesn't want to do them and I do them.' Similarly a mother talking of her daughter's problem in finding a job and then keeping it for more than a couple of days said: 'so I helped her to get a small job just down the road'. When this did not last long either this mother's reaction was: 'as long as she's busy down at the day centre I don't mind'. Another mother describing her well-educated son's efforts to start work again said: 'If he can get going with a part-time job (cleaning in a theatre) it'll get him back into the routine.'

Deviant behaviour could not always be removed but it could be limited. Some successful relatives adopted rules; for example, 'listen to voices only in the bedroom', or 'no talking to himself at mealtimes'. If delusions or hallucinations became very prominent, such relatives learned that it was not helpful to try to argue the patient out of them since this only made matters worse. Instead, these relatives had learned to accept that the delusion was real enough to the patient. A father described saying to his son: 'your experiences are real, but only to you'. Another relative called it 'meeting it halfway', i.e. she would agree about its reality to the patient but tried to reassure him. If someone thought that a knob in the wall was a hidden microphone this mother said she would 'take it to pieces and show it to him'. Alternatively comforting someone might help: 'there's no one there, hold on to me and it will go away'. Another useful strategy for difficult behaviour was to divert attention on to something else. When a son said he hated his work one morning, his mother did not reply but just asked him what he wanted for breakfast. He later went to work as usual. An approach this mother also used with her 35-year-old son was to take it lightly.'If he won't get up in the morning I make a joke of it, I say: "Head or feet first?" and then I pull his feet down to the mat on the floor.'

An integral part of this neutral but supportive reaction seems to be the ability to stay calm oneself. One father whose son suddenly announced a mission to kill him said, 'It didn't worry me. I thought: "If he goes for me I'll put him in his place" . . . I wasn't too upset though, as the wife had a breakdown once . . . I do take things as they come I suppose.' In a similar incident a wife described how her husband came up to her with a kitchen knife and asked her to kill him. She replied, 'No I don't want to kill you'; this defused the situation, they were able to talk about it and he put the knife down. A less dramatic example was when a wife talked of her husband's complete refusal to get up, even to wash for a few days after he had had some teeth out. She said: 'I didn't push it; I didn't lose my temper but just asked him to get up once each day and then left it . . . He got up and dressed'. This sort of controlled response appears related to the ability to separate illness-related behaviour from what is seen as aspects of the personality.

In the most recent research, two-thirds of the critical remarks seemed to be related to behaviour that relatives felt had always been there and had always been disliked. No allowance or understanding was therefore given to it being due to an illness, which could be seen as less provocative and deliberate, and for which allowances could be made. Critical relatives insisted that patients had *always* been like it: 'She's been petty and selfish and spoilt since she was little', said one father about his daughter, and a daughter said about her mother who complained of hearing voices, 'it didn't cut no ice with me, there's nothing really *mentally* wrong'.

It is very hard to change long-felt opinions about someone or to stop being irritated by something, some habit or piece of behaviour. Some people do annoy each other, and this is particularly obvious in families. Fortunately, as well as finding differences between critical and non-critical relatives, a number of other ways of coping were found to be helpful to patients which involved less radical changes in the attitudes of relatives.

Two factors were found to be helpful in keeping a patient well even if he returned to live in a critical rather than a non-critical family: first, staying on the prescribed medication; second, having a restricted amount of face-to-face contact with the highly critical or over-involved relative. It is now well established that phenothiazine medication is one of the most efficient ways of controlling the more disruptive symptoms of a psychotic illness such as schizophrenia. Because it can only control symptoms rather than cure the underlying predisposition, medication often has to be taken for some years. In this sense schizophrenia can be likened to a disease such as diabetes, where daily injections of insulin are necessary to maintain a healthy state. Although daily tablets can be replaced by injections, which last two to four weeks, many patients still object to being under constant medication and therefore discontinue it. One objection is to the side-effects, another is the dislike of having to depend on drugs, a third is a difficulty in understanding that medication should be continued even when the patient is feeling well.

The other protective factor is to cut down contact with a highly critical relative. Some patients discover this for themselves. For instance one man reversed his day; he got up at night when the rest of the family was asleep, and slept during the day. Other ways of reducing contact are for the patient to spend his days out of the house at a job or at a day centre. This is not always possible, of course, because it is hard to obtain employment, or because there is a lack of day centres, or because the patient refuses to go to one. Alternatives are for the relatives themselves to find work or spend time out of the house. Actually spending time in the same room, 'face to face', is the situation to be avoided. In some cases it is possible for patient and critical relative to spend time in different rooms, even in the same house. As one retired father said about his son: 'when he gets bad I shut myself in my room and attend to my own affairs'. Other possibilities if the relatives are parents is for the son or daughter to be encouraged to leave home altogether and try living in some form of sheltered accommodation such as a hostel. Again, there is a lack of hostel places, and some patients and relatives, particularly those with the most intense and involved relationships, refuse to live apart like that. However, it can be seen as a way of encouraging independence and separate interests for all concerned, and can help relieve the final worry of ageing parents, of who will look after the patient when they are gone.

The theoretical reasons for strategies such as reduced face-to-face contact, and a calm and detached response to disturbed behaviour are probably connected to ideas about the inability of schizophrenics to take in too much stimulation at one time. This may be because they are more physiologically aroused than other people or because they are more confused and are limited in what they can take in. One acutely ill schizophrenic patient said: 'when people talk to me it's like a different sort of language. It's too much to hold at once' and 'I can't concentrate, it's a diversion of attention that troubles me—the sounds are coming through to me but I feel my mind cannot cope with everything'. An intrusive or emotional relationship adds to such difficulties.

Given that, for whatever reasons, some reactions of relatives and some methods of coping seem to be more helpful than others when living with a mentally ill person, the question arises as to how best to help those families who cope least well and who are, concomitantly, the most upset and the most liable to be faced with hospital readmissions, with all the disturbances leading up to and surrounding these. Work has been done trying to offer help to families in this position, mainly offering help with specific problems that they face. However, the most noticeable feature of such work is how many of the families drop out of such treatment—do not carry on coming to the sessions or therapy, or who prefer to be left alone. One reason seems to be a disillusion with professional help, particularly over the course of a long illness when professionals have patently been unable to help. As a result such families often feel very isolated, feel they suffer from lack of information about what was going to happen to them, and frequently complain of a lack of coordinated services and advice as to the best way of managing. These feelings are undoubtedly due, at least in part, to a genuine failure on the part of professionals who, in turn, often feel at a loss in the face of long-term illness. They may also be unaware of the specialist knowledge that is only just becoming available. One way round this is to help relatives who live with the mentally ill to help each other, since those who do manage well are potentially in an ideal position to share their solutions with others with the same problems. This sort of work is just beginning to be done and evaluated, and the second part of the chapter gives an account of one such group of relatives which is already functioning.

The knowledge recently gained should also be useful to those who work in residential settings and day centres, who also need to learn from relatives how to 'live with schizophrenia' so that patients are helped to become as independent as possible.

PART II. Helping a self-help group

The National Schizophrenia Fellowship is one of the many self-help organizations that have developed during the past ten years, more or less consciously based on the model of similar bodies earlier established to foster the welfare of people with physical illnesses or disabilities such as diabetes or spasticity or multiple sclerosis. In the case of schizophrenia, the need for such a body illustrates with special clarity the isolation that families feel because of rejecting community attitudes and the lack of effective supporting health and social services. Creer and Wing showed that relatives who joined the Fellowship were those who had experienced particularly difficult problems and this should be remembered when reading the rest of this chapter. The other special factor concerns the nature of the diagnosis of schizophrenia. This is usually based on the presence of the highly specific symptoms described earlier. Sometimes, however, the term 'schizophrenia' is used in a looser way, to designate conditions of severe social disablement which seem to have no explanation, even though specific symptoms have never been present. Both groups of conditions are disabling and distressing, and relatives need a great deal of help, but they may not respond to precisely the same methods of treatment or counselling. The first part of this chapter was concerned with schizophrenia narrowly defined. Here we are dealing with a much more diverse range of conditions.

The author, a professional nurse and social administrator, was appointed in 1976 by the National Schizophrenia Fellowship, in order to act as an intermediary between a locally organized group of relatives and the statutory services. The work resolved itself naturally into two parts: first, to identify and help to meet needs for services; second, to foster the resources that existed within the local group of relatives. The first of these problems is dealt with in more detail in other chapters and I shall concentrate chiefly upon the second.

The need for information

A survey of the problems experienced by relatives showed that one of the principal complaints was that little advice was given on specific difficulties of 'management'. Questions on such subjects were ignored by professional advisers or answered unhelpfully. The group of relatives I was concerned with rarely asked the psychiatrist what the diagnosis meant but some did look it up in out-of-date encyclopaedias in the public library, obtaining some useless technical jargon but no enlightenment.

Lack of advice about how the services work or where to turn for help added to the confusion and emotional exhaustion of psychiatric patients and their families. Facts about welfare benefits, compulsory admission, emergency help, social and work rehabilitation, accommodation, and voluntary support were not easily available. It was not uncommon for relatives to seek help from Citizens Advice Bureaux or the Samaritans, but these agencies were not well-placed to give the help needed. There are disadvantages in giving printed information about such a complex range of services, since it quickly becomes out of date and services are so unevenly distributed that the facility needed is often lacking or inaccessible. Ideally, service information should be made available in the context of an informed counselling service, readily available to relatives and patients and acceptable to them because they have been consulted as to how it should be set up. This means that problems of personal relationships between patient and relatives can also be dealt with. Any family coping with a chronic illness at home needs continuous support from someone who is known and trusted. Should this come from the family doctor, the social worker, a community nurse, or an experienced volunteer?

The traditional relationship between professional and relative is one that sometimes seems to require dependence. The doctor or nurse may expect or be expected to answer questions or provide prescriptive advice, because of the authoritative nature of the consultation. If there are no immediate rules on how to cope with psychotic or withdrawn behaviour the professional adviser may feel helpless and may, as a result, appear abrupt, even aggressive. The relative may then withdraw from any further questions about very real and distressing problems. The relationship needs to be changed to one of mutual learning and contributions to possible solutions. This demands from professionals the capacity to empathize, to put themselves into the shoes of the relative or patient in order to understand what the problems are and to enable them to take an active part in finding ways of relieving stressful situations. Premature advice, given without allowing time for all parties to define the problem, may be felt as patronizing and unrealistic. Training in counselling should help to correct traditional professional perspectives.

This may seem very obvious but it is only too clear that many health and social service workers are unable to really listen or understand, partly because of their need to provide answers. Moreover, many are not aware of the body of work outlined in the first part of this chapter. Similarly, relatives may be unable to talk freely because of the formality of the relationship. One relative expressed something like this when she said how helpful it had been to have psychiatrists and other professionals visiting a relatives' group because it was the only time when they could meet 'on neutral ground', and this provided a unique experience. The implication is that help or support is needed which is unrestricted by the standard professional consultancy role.

The role of a professional worker in a self-help group

There are now many types of self-help groups, each with its own more or less defined set of goals. It seems clear that the main factor is that all groups share the experience of a particular problem, which can be made available to all group-members, often on a trial-and-error basis. The role of a professional is therefore to promote mutual empathy, support and peer learning, without creating dependence and without taking over the responsibility for exercising skills which the members should exercise for themselves.

The following account describes an attempt to act as an enabler to a local group of the National Schizophrenia Fellowship, which consisted of approximately 100 members at the time of the study. The majority of these members were parents of a schizophrenic son or daughter. In five areas of 'Southshire', house group meetings took place every other month in the homes of relatives. These afforded members the opportunity to meet others with similar experiences, to talk about their problems in a way which would be impossible elsewhere, and to find opportunities for mutual support. It is not uncommon for a family coping with mental illness at home to become totally isolated and resigned to a life of sacrifice and strain. One mother in a group meeting said: 'We have become used to accepting the abnormal as normal.' This is a common reaction of families containing a severely handicapped member and is by no means confined to schizophrenia, but relatives are not to know that.

The attendance at these group meetings was very erratic to start with, and I proposed that I should work closely with a new group of relatives, in order to look more closely at what was happening. It was agreed that I should work with one new group for a limited period of time and that it would remain essentially a self-help group which might develop into an action group with its own leadership. My role would be a facilitating one, both inside and outside the group. It was agreed that fortnightly meetings would present opportunities for solidarity and for observing patterns of behaviour and adaptation.

To bring together a group which has no agreed task and is not a therapeutic group throws a great strain on the group leader. However, in this situation to define the task would be to define the problems in advance. The self-help group needs to define its own problems which may be different from those expected by professionals. My own aims were as follows:

1. To provide a focus for the group, which was for the relatives to gain more insight through each other and to share information and experiences. In particular to explore how to cope with dependency and intense emotional involvement.

2. To provide or clarify information needed to make the most of available services.

3. To invite local professionals, representing different services, to attend occasional open sessions.

4. To encourage interaction and mutual support outside the group.

5. To follow-up, with the relevant services, those families which clearly indicated an inadequacy of support which could be rectified within the limits of available services.

6. To try to foster such a degree of awareness in the group, or in a substantial sub-group, that my own role would become redundant.

Group membership

It was not feasible, within a voluntary organization, to have many rules about membership and attendance. Ideally, the membership of the group should be not less than 6 or more than 12, and it was hoped that members would feel committed to regular attendance if any continuity or cohesion was to develop. When a hard core of members have got to know each other it becomes easier to accommodate a new member. If there are constant changes it is likely that the group will not survive, or that the members who have attended regularly will find the procedure repetitive and stressful.

The following account is based on 20 fortnightly sessions with this group, over a period of 10 months. A total of 25 members of the Fellowship living in one locality were invited to attend at some point. Fourteen of these members were married couples. Twenty of those invited attended on one or more occasions. Of these, eleven became a central core group by attending regularly and expressing commitment to continuing membership in future. Several months of irregular attendance elapsed before this commitment was made. Of these eleven members, seven are mothers and two are fathers. The other two are women committed to the group as members of the Southshire Committee. One has experience as the wife of a schizophrenic man, the other as the friend of a man who committed suicide. Two married couples attend together. Two of the mothers are single parents with daughters. A son and two daughters have each attended for one session.

Venue of the group

The fact that most relatives' groups run by Fellowship members take place in private homes, providing an apparently 'neutral ground', may be very important. For our group, the use of a day centre for the mentally ill was requested from the Social Services Department. The reasons for this were threefold. First, it might enable the voluntary organization to make itself known to the services and claim more support from them. Second, it provided comfortable, homely surroundings, unlike many other public buildings. Third, it provided an easily accessible centre for those using public transport.

The group members expressed mixed feelings. They felt that they were less likely to be 'taken over' if they met in each others' homes. On the other hand, not all of them could offer accommodation and the onus tended to fall on one person, who necessarily became a sort of leader in the group. In fact, the day centre provided a convenient and reliable central point and encouraged a commitment to turn up.

If a viable, autonomous group is to develop it seems vital that professional staff should respect its independence and not attend meetings unless invited to do so. The presence of observers in such groups, however sympathetic, would change the entire nature of the meeting. The members would be reacting, however unconsciously, to the presence of the intruder. A group where members of hospital staff and relatives meet together to exchange information and ideas on management can be very helpful to both parties but it should be organized separately.

Leadership style

It was clear that a major part of the study of this group would involve observing the effect of my own presence. Incidents had been reported of other Fellowship relatives' groups where members had felt that social workers did not understand their problems, or made them feel guilty, or led them to feel they were being studied. My position might have been made easier by the fact that I was a professional employed by the Fellowship itself and that I did not, therefore, represent part of the 'system'.

In the early stages the members repeatedly tested my reactions to their anger and resentment of the 'experts'. If I had allied myself with the experts this anger and frustration would have had no outlet. Alternatively, if I continued to reinforce or confirm the validity of their complaints a point could not be reached where they could make use of each other to look for positive solutions. It is important for anyone in the position of group leader to be aware of the nature of their own involvement and to understand what is happening in terms of both individual and group behaviour. Bearing in mind that my role in this group was to bring about my own redundancy if possible, my approach was as non-directive as was possible without arousing anxiety or frustration. My function was to confront, clarify, and contain, and these three functions are considered in more detail below. I also initiated discussions, acted as time-keeper, encouraged diffident members, and answered direct questions as best I could. Interpretations of group and individual behaviour were limited to 'here-and-now' observations, particularly of a need to place me into a position of authority, and to discuss technical rather than personal problems. As members became more confident I was able to relinquish some of the leadership role.

(i) Confrontation

Confrontation might involve bringing into sharp relief a piece of behaviour from a relative's account of problems at home. For example, a mother lays a place for her daughter at the breakfast table and prepares the meal for her every morning. The daughter then refuses to eat. If the mother does not make these preparations, she is convinced her daughter will not bother to get anything for herself and will starve. The procedure has become a kind of game between them and the circle has to be broken. The interpretation that her need to feed her daughter may be greater than her daughter's determination to starve is not made directly. My part here would be to allow other relatives to identify the situation and suggest to the mother alternative ways of coping.

It is clear that relatives have applied a wide range of techniques in order to prevent stress at home. If this results in both the patient and the relative feeling better it has been successful. If the cost to the relative is rigid control of her own feelings it has not been successful. The patient is likely to be very sensitive to such control. When these adaptations are discussed it becomes possible for some relatives, because of the reactions of others, to appreciate the situation. For example, a daughter was using and misusing her mother's personal possessions. To avoid a scene, the mother suppressed her feelings of irritation and annoyance. She developed a recurring headache. One morning she intuitively felt her restraint was wrong and, in an outburst of anger, she told her daughter that she wanted her possessions left alone. There was no scene, her daughter obeyed, and seemed almost relieved. By the evening the headache had gone. No interpretation from the group leader was necessary. All the work was done by members of the group, who had been through similar experiences themselves.

(ii) Clarification

Clarification has often been necessary about the nature of schizophrenia and its treatment and prognosis. Relatives have needed a great deal of help in understanding that this is not a clearly defined illness with a specific form of treatment. Clarification is also needed in explaining how the services work or do not work. For example, a relative may feel very neglected because no social worker has been to see the family following the patient's discharge from hospital. They may not know that no referral from the hospital has been made. It has to be pointed out that many families are known about, but social services remain unable to offer the kind of counselling support which is needed, because of lack of resources and professional training. This is the fact and relatives have to accept it. One of the functions of a body such as the National Schizophrenia Fellowship is to bring such facts to the attention of the authorities and to suggest remedies.

Another area where clarification is needed is in helping relatives to separate practical from emotional issues. Guilt and a great need to make some recompense for the tragedy of this condition can lead relatives to see the schizophrenic patient as a child in need of constant protection. They may long to go on holiday and resent being tied but be unable to leave a son or daughter alone. Even when the realistic fears are dealt with, they may still be unwilling to give up a nursing role. Other relatives can be helpful by offering practical help, such as keeping an eye on a son or daughter left alone, and also emotional support in understanding their fears of what might happen. The boundary between what is a proper and responsible concern for a handicapped person, and what is an overprotective response that leads to unnecessary dependency, is very difficult to draw. The group counsellor has to try to keep a reasonable balance.

There are aspects of living with psychotics which are unique, such as coping with delusions. Much of the reported behaviour which causes disruption and stress in home life is analogous to behaviour in a very difficult child who has become omnipotent and manipulates his or her family. If relatives can understand the difficulty a schizophrenic person has in seeing himself or herself as a separate identity then they can begin to help to make the boundaries clear. The mother with the daughter who messed up her things finally had to say, 'These are my possessions, not yours'. The mother who made her daughter's break-fast every morning needed to say, 'Please get yourself some breakfast if you want it'. People with schizophrenia may show childlike behaviour but they are not children and the problems are correspondingly dif-ficult to cope with. Some relatives go to the other extreme of denying that disability exists; they have completely unrealistic expectations. The group experience acts as a corrective in both types of situation.

(iii) Containment

Reporting intensely painful and sometimes intractable problems can cause a great deal of anxiety in such a group. A relative who has not been able to talk to anyone about his or her problems can drain and exhaust others. The usual physical kind of comforting that takes place between friends may seem inappropriate. The emotion then gets denied or 'patted away'. The upset member needs understanding and acceptance of powerful emotions. If the other members can allow feelings to be expressed and share the experience with the relative the anxiety can often be released. The leader is expected to contain this level of anxiety, to make it safe, to prevent chaos, but the real suppor-ters are those members of the group who have learned through their own personal experience that it *is* possible to live through very painful and harrowing scenes without losing their own sense of identity and balance. The leader has to bring out this healthy reaction.

The process of the group

The tools for recording and assessing the process of what actually happens in such a group are inadequate. I shall try to illustrate some examples of exchanges between relatives, in order to show the pos-sibilities for support, behaviour modification and healthy attitude change. In my introduction to the group I emphasized that this was a collaborative venture between relatives and myself, to look at the problems of management of a schizophrenic condition. Three themes or preoccupations were constantly emerging and deserve separate discussion: 'What is schizophrenia?'; 'The services are bad and the "experts" do not understand or help'; 'How can a son or daughter be helped to achieve an optimum level of contentment and independence?'

(i) What is schizophrenia?

I have found it helpful, if asked a direct question, to use the introductory chapter to the Fellowship booklet—*Schizophrenia from within*. This looks at the meaning of the illness in terms of the patient's own experiences and is sceptical about various theories of causation, in view of the lack of hard evidence. In view of the wide range of conditions that are called 'schizophrenic' (and it is this diagnosis that leads the relative to join the Fellowship), I have found it useful to ask, first, what the relative understands by the term schizophrenia. In this way the fantasies of incurability, madness, violence, and total dependence can be brought out into the open and looked at by other relatives in a supportive way. The way in which a relative perceives 'schizophrenia' may profoundly affect the way in which he or she responds to it. For example, a parent may have a deep conviction that in some way the illness is his or her fault, and will prepare for a life of devoted sacrifice which could be detrimental to recovery. This kind of attitude is reinforced by the theories of some fashionable pundits and it cannot be simply contradicted. Again, the experience of the group can help to bring about a more balanced attitude.

(ii) The services are inadequate

Of course, the services *are* inadequate. We have had psychiatrists, a social worker, a nurse, a voluntary worker and a Disablement Resettlement Officer, visit the group, and this may have helped in a small way to increase understanding and open two-way communication. I have intervened on behalf of relatives when it seems that some available service is not being offered or when members of the group seemed to have a wrong impression of what was available.

As with the first topic it is necessary to be aware of the way in which a group can use the subject of 'bashing experts' as a diversionary activity. A self-help group can achieve its cohesion by a feeling of banding together against a common enemy. This may well present a force for change in a group which is seeking political action, but there is a danger of negative and unconstructive bitterness. The complaints of relatives are legitimate. They receive very inadequate support. Factual information about services can help them to improve the situation and to be more aware of the kind of support available. It can also leave them resentful and despairing, when a service that they ought to be able to rely on is not available. This emotion can be used in a positive way by bringing political pressure to bear. This is another role of the Fellowship, and deserves support from professional people.

(iii) How can someone with schizophrenia be helped to achieve an optimum level of contentment and independence?

An attempt was made in our group to focus on strengthening the personal resources of relatives. They were encouraged to examine in detail what goes on at home and to compare this with the problems of others. In this way they learned a great deal, as the following examples demonstrate.

(a). A relative pointed out that a father's resistance to his daughter entering hospital ('that terrible place') had more to do with his own fear than that of his daughter. Relatives who had experienced this 'horror' themselves, and found the hospital quite helpful, encouraged him to consider his attitudes to hospital, which might be prejudiced.

(b). Relatives pointed out to a mother that she was being over-protective to her daughter and suggested the daughter get a job. Those who were previously themselves most over-protective were the most vociferous in pointing this out.

(c). A relative disagreed with a father who strongly denied his daughter's delusions, telling her they were 'rubbish'. This relative learned to understand that a delusion is reality to a schizophrenic patient, but also to keep separate his own knowledge that the belief was a false one. The same father asked the group's advice about 'giving in' to his daughter and agreed about the possibility that he had been 'over-pampering'.

(d). A mother who had been very depressed, and spoke in a quiet, whining voice, was able to say that she felt sometimes that she could kill her daughter. The other mothers identified with this, implying it was not such an unnatural feeling in the circumstances. All present found that they could laugh, even about such topics, a release that all those who care for the handicapped require from time to time.

Conclusions

No criteria have yet been established to define the success or failure of a venture of this kind. It can be assumed that the eleven existing members have 'voted with their feet' on the issue of the continuation of the group, with or without my own leadership. There is a lively interest, at this point, in helping to develop a further self-help group composed of the patients themselves.

The irregular attendance at this group during the first months made it very difficult to develop any solidarity or purpose. It was not until the last two months that cohesion and some sense of autonomy emerged. The members expressed a wish for continuing leadership from outside. They wanted someone who was 'an anchor' or a 'catalyst' who would allow them to continue the present structure of the group. To this extent, my original aim, to make myself redundant, was not fulfilled, and it is not clear that a natural leader will emerge from the group itself. Moreover, the function of acting as an intermediary with the existing services does need some professional expertise.

Self-help groups have a potential for helping those living with severe mental illness which statutory services cannot hope to provide—the release from isolation and feelings of stigma offered by a community of people who share similar experiences. The link between these groups and the mental health services is a vital one if the patient is not to be treated in isolation. The standard lay–professional relationship therefore needs to be modified. The most important factor in the helping process in this group was personal experience of the problems. Relatives were much more able to accept suggestions and criticisms from each other than from a professional worker. A second vital factor was that support was ongoing rather than episodic.

The role of a professional in a group which uses self-help principles needs to be enabling and facilitating, so that resources within the group can be mobilized. A doctor, a nurse, a social worker, or a counsellor, might equally well run such a group if they had the ability to use their own personal resources of warmth and empathy, as well as relying on their professional expertise. Above all, they should be able to learn from the experience of patients and relatives. If they do not have these personal resources, or if there is a professional rigidity in their relationship with others, they will neither be able to learn from those they see as needing professional advice, nor be able to help liberate them from restrictive attitudes.

The experience with this group has convinced me that it is possible for professional people to work creatively with relatives to reduce disability and distress.

FURTHER READING

Brown, G. W., Bone, M., Dalison, B. and Wing, J. K. (1966). *Schizophrenia and social care*. Oxford University Press, London.

Creer, C. and Wing, J. K. (1974). *Schizophrenia at home*. National Schizophrenia Fellowship, 78 Victoria Road, Surbiton, Surrey KT6 4JT.

Hirsch, S. R. and Leff, J. P. (1975). *Abnormalities in parents of schizophrenics: a review of the literature and an investigation of communication aspects and deviances*. Oxford University Press, London.

National Schizophrenia Fellowship (1974). *Living with schizophrenics: by the relatives*. National Schizophrenia Fellowship, 78 Victoria Road, Surbiton, Surrey KT6 4JT.
Vaughn, C. E. and Leff, J. P. (1976). The influence of family and social factors on the course of psychiatric illness. *Br. J. Psychiat*. **129**, 125–37.
Wing, J. K. (ed.) (1975). *Schizophrenia from within*. National Schizophrenia Fellowship, 78 Victoria Road, Surbiton, Surrey KT6 4JT.
— (ed.) (1978). *Schizophrenia: towards a new synthesis*. Academic Press, London.
— and Brown, G. W. (1970).
Institutionalism and schizophrenia. Cambridge University Press, London.

3 Day services and the mentally ill

Carol Edwards and Jan Carter

On any given day, 15 000 people attend about 400 day units for the mentally ill in England and Wales.[1] These day units are in settings of many types and sizes, and they play an important part in extending the spectrum of care and treatment available for people suffering from mental illness. In view of the trends discussed in Chapter 1, day care can be expected to play an ever-increasing role.

The purposes of this chapter are twofold: first to give a descriptive account of the day services which authorities provide for adults who have had the experience of mental illness, and second by comparing the services of the major providers—area health authorities and social services departments—to question why separate services exist and what the implications are for the people who attend.

Who provides day services, and why?

There are three major providers of day services for the mentally ill in England and Wales: the National Health Service through local area health authorities (AHA), local authority social services departments (SSD), and voluntary organizations. These divisions between AHA and SSD provision are reflected in government policy, and are one feature of the network of district services envisaged by the government's policy statement of 1975. This White Paper proposed that the AHA day hospitals should have 'facilities for treatment . . . for group and individual therapy. It should also provide a wide range of occupational and rehabilitation activities'. Although the White Paper ack-

<hr>

[1] Estimates in this chapter are based on 1976 figures collected during a national survey which investigated day services for all adult user groups in thirteen local authorities of England and Wales. The research was financed by the Joseph Rowntree Memorial Trust, and a full publication of the results is being prepared. The local authorities, day units, staff, and attenders who participated in the survey were all chosen by sampling procedures described in the full publication. Forty day units for the mentally ill participated in the survey. Of these, twenty AHA day hospitals, seven SSD day centres, and two voluntary centres were included in the interview sample, from which 394 interviews were collected, 178 with attenders and 116 with those who worked in the units.

nowledged that it was difficult to draw an exact line between the functions of SSD day centres and AHA day hospitals, one goal of SSD day centres was 'to meet clients' immediate needs for shelter, occupation, and social activity. In so doing, the centre may also serve to relieve the strain on the client's family.' Day centres were to 'help with difficulties in forming or maintaining personal relationships . . . adjusting or readjusting to the demands of work . . . [and to] encourage the realization of the individual's potential'. Basically, the paper specified that the 'social' aspects of care could be emphasized by day centres, while the more 'medical' aspects could be conducted in day hospitals. But a very large area of overlap persisted—particularly inasmuch as both services were recommended as places to keep attenders occupied.

The White Paper also gave planning guidelines for day places: there should be 0.3 day hospital places, and 0.6 day centre places, per 1000 population. The national survey found that each of the thirteen areas, defined by local authority/health authority boundaries, had at least one AHA day hospital, but only about half had a SSD day centre. On average, one forty-place day hospital served a population of about 200 000, which was well below the government guideline of 0.3 day hospital places per 1000 population. However, there was some extra concentration of day places in AHAs in London. Because of the size of some of the areas, the actual distance to be travelled to the nearest day hospital could be very large. The SSD day centres, which were somewhat smaller than day hospitals (they had 33 day places on average), were also more concentrated in London boroughs than elsewhere in the country, and where they existed at all in an authority there was most likely only one. Thus day centre places fell even further than day hospital places below their planning ratio of 0.6 day centre places per 1000 population.

The fact that AHAs are the largest providers of day services, sponsoring about three-quarters of all day units for the mentally ill whereas the SSDs provide only a fifth, is related to the history of their development. In 1946 the first British day hospital (the 'Social Psychotherapy Centre', later the Marlborough Day Hospital) was opened in London. The number of day hospitals for the mentally ill open in the 1950s had roughly tripled by the 1960s, and this number had doubled again by 1975. SSD day centres have a shorter history than day hospitals: nearly all of them have opened during the seventies, and thus have not had time to achieve parity of numbers with AHA provision. However, if each service continued to expand at the present rate, the amount of SSD provision would remain behind AHA provision instead of overtaking it.

The national survey indicated that about a quarter of AHA day hospitals were located outside hospital sites. Most of these were in self-contained premises near the local high street or business district, or in residential areas; the rest shared premises with other establishments such as health clinics. The majority of day hospitals, however, were located in the grounds or on the premises of hospitals. Over a third, for example, already operated within the new district general hospitals as government policy recommended, taking their place alongside the other out-patient and in-patient psychiatric services available there. Another third were scattered around the country in the grounds of the large psychiatric hospitals. Some of these day hospitals were situated within the hospital buildings themselves, for example occupying a former in-patient ward.

According to a third of the day hospital workers interviewed in 1976, one aim of the day hospitals was to keep people out of psychiatric hospital. Clinically assessing day patients and providing treatment for their disorders was mentioned by over a quarter, and an equal number emphasized the importance of the eventual return of patients to independent life in the community.[2] All three aims reiterate those envisaged by the government policy paper of 1975.

The second largest providers of day services, the local authority social services departments, call their units 'centres' rather than 'hospitals'. Day centres were never situated in hospitals, but were occasionally attached to hostels. Their aims, as expressed by those who worked in the centres, were found to differ significantly from those of day hospitals in only two respects: the idea that the day centre should clinically assess and treat people was absent, but instead a quarter of the staff said the day centre aimed to provide a range of concrete, practical services to the people who attend, such as a meal and the company of other people.

The area of overlap already mentioned between centres and hospitals was demonstrated by the similar proportion of people working in both sectors who mentioned the aim of keeping people out of hospital and re-establishing them outside.

The third type of day service for the mentally ill is provided by voluntary organizations. First in the field is MIND: the National Association for Mental Health. Local MIND groups run various services for people with mental illness which also seek to involve lonely and isolated people. Most of these services run for a couple of hours a

---

[2] Detailed information about the aims of day units is contained in the final reports of the national survey, currently in preparation.

week, often on a club basis, and include such groups as social clubs, handicraft clubs, and therapeutic clubs. But for the purposes of the national survey, a day unit as opposed to a club had to be open at least fifteen hours a week over at least three days. Two local MIND groups did run day centres in the study areas which met this minimum requirement. In fact both exceeded it, staying open on Saturday and Sunday and many evenings as well. However, not many voluntary groups in the country are able to offer such a lengthy service each week. These voluntary day centres comprised only about 5 per cent of the total number of units available to mentally ill people in England and Wales. Because of this, and since the sample of voluntary day centres surveyed was so small, their contribution will be mentioned only when it seems particularly pertinent.

Who participates in day services?

There are two groups of people in day units: the men and women who attend the day unit, called 'users', and the people employed to work in the day unit, called the 'staff'. In individual units users are called 'clients', 'patients', or occasionally members of the day unit. Staff are usually named by their job description as 'nurse', 'instructor', etc. Various names are given to the person with responsibility for the day-to-day running of the day unit, and these were simplified into the appellation 'head'. In SSD day centres this person was usually the officer-in-charge or manager, and in AHA day hospitals he or she was the nursing officer, sister-in-charge, or charge nurse. For the purposes of the survey the nurses were regarded as heads, instead of consultants or senior registrars who hold formal clinical responsibility for day hospital patients, since they usually spent all their time in the day hospital and their work more closely paralleled the work of day centre managers.

Who are the users?
Nearly two hundred users who were attending day units for the mentally ill in thirteen areas of England and Wales were interviewed in 1976. There were slightly more men attending SSD day centres than women, whereas in AHA day hospitals there were more women than men, though in both the margin was not very wide. In SSD day centres the users ranged in age from 20 to 78, with an average age of 46 years, but the largest group were in their thirties. The range of ages in day hospitals was similar to that in day centres, and although the average age in day hospitals (41 years) was somewhat younger than the average

in day centres, the largest group of attenders in day hospitals were in their fifties. There was an equal proportion of married and single people in the day hospitals—the married people usually lived with their spouses, while those who were single tended to live alone or with their parents. Only a very small proportion lived in a hospital or other sheltered residential accommodation. The pattern for users of SSD day centres was very similar, though they were more likely to be single than married, and more lived alone or in hospitals, hostels, or lodgings than their peers in AHA day hospitals.

Differences between the ways that users perceived their own physical and mental health in AHA day hospitals and SSD day centres were slight. About four-fifths of the users, attending either type of unit, described a current mental or emotional disorder. For these people the administrative label for the day unit as being 'for the mentally ill' seemed to match their perception of their own difficulties. The rest, one-fifth, fell into two small groups. Half described a physical complaint such as heart trouble, a circulatory disease or the like, while the other half did not consider that they had either a current mental or a current physical disorder. One should remember that this information reflects the user's own perception of his health, and as such does not necessarily conform either with a medical diagnosis or with the perception of a user's health held by family or friends. Although it was not possible to substantiate the validity of this information by an independent assessment of each individual's disorder, a check was made of the consistency with which users who named a mental disorder described symptoms within the last month of anxiety, nervousness, irrational fears, sleeplessness, etc. This was compared to those who did not name a mental disorder. In both day centres and day hospitals users naming a mental disorder tended to describe more recent symptoms, on average, than those who said they were without a mental disorder.[3] This indicates a degree of internal consistency in the users' reports of their own conditions, although obviously a possible underestimation of disorder compared to the views of their doctors.

A closer look at the nature of problems described by people with mental or emotional disorders again showed striking similarities between the descriptions of those in SSD and AHA day units. About half in both types of units described their condition in terms of their symptoms, without reference to any diagnostic label: for example, 'nerves', 'mental strain', and 'unable to cope with pressure' were

[3] Reports of recent symptoms of anxiety, nervousness, irrational fears, etc., were twice as common among users in units for the mentally ill compared to units for other user groups such as the physically handicapped or elderly.

mentioned. About a third in AHA day hospitals and a fifth in SSD day centres called their disorder 'depression'. About another fifth of the people in SSD units (17 per cent) said they suffered from schizophrenia or manic depression—this was double the proportion who mentioned these conditions in AHA units.

One extension to this information about mental disorders was possible in relation to depression. The users who *labelled* their condition as depression indicated almost without exception that they *felt* depressed too. However, many more users than the third in day hospitals and the fifth in day centres who called their disorder depression admitted to feeling depressed. In fact, two-thirds of the 178 users interviewed said they had felt depressed (that is, 'unhappy, in low spirits, downcast, or gloomy') in the last month. Four out of five of the people who had felt depressed also felt like committing suicide. From their descriptions of how often they felt depressed and how long the depression lasted it was possible to assess the severity of the condition as experienced by the user. It was here that there were some differences between SSD and AHA attenders, for more users in AHA day hospitals had been feeling depressed in the last month. Also, more of their descriptions of depression were rated by an independent researcher and a psychiatrist as 'moderate' or 'considerable' than users in SSD day centres. In fact, over half the users in day hospitals were rated as 'moderately' or 'considerably' depressed. This included depression experienced with some regularity (at least once a week) and which lasted for part of the day and depression which lasted for days at a time without relief. 'Moderate' or 'considerable' depression was experienced by about two-fifths of users in SSD day centres. Thus there seemed to be some tendency for people who felt depressed to be in AHA day hospitals rather than in SSD day centres.

The extent to which users had previously made use of some psychiatric services was also assessed. For four out of five day hospital users this was their first experience of day as opposed to in-patient services, since they had not attended any other day unit for the mentally ill. But over half said they had lived for some time in psychiatric hospitals: about a fifth for a year or more. The SSD users were more experienced consumers of day and in-patient psychiatric services than their AHA peers. About half said they had attended at least one, and sometimes two or three, day units before. Three-quarters said they had lived in a psychiatric hospital, and in five out ten cases this was for a year or more. So more SSD users had lived in psychiatric hospital than AHA users and for longer periods, which suggests that there is more chronic psychiatric disability among SSD users. In voluntary sponsored units the past psychiatric service experiences of users were more similar to the experiences of the majority of SSD users than to AHA users.

The impression of lengthy usage of psychiatric services was reinforced by the length of time users had attended day services. Day services may have been a new experience for the majority of users initially, but by the time of the survey many of them had been coming for a long time. Over half of those in SSD day centres and voluntary sponsored units, and a third in AHA day hospitals, had been attending for a year or more (in fact, one in three of this long-stay group had attended for over five years). This information parallels the findings of other research which suggests there is a build-up of long-stay users in day services. When ex-patients are discharged from psychiatric hospitals as part of the run-down of long-stay beds, many appear to be finding their way into day units, and there embark on another long term of attendance.

An inspection of the actual number of users discharged from day units each year adds a further dimension. The greater build-up of long-stay users in day centres is related not only to the greater chronicity of some users but also to the fact that day centres discharge a smaller number of users each year in comparison to day hospitals. While the day centres surveyed each discharged 28 users a year, the day hospitals each discharged 86 users, on average. However, this information gives no account of how many, say, of the 86 users discharged came back to the day hospital later in the year.[4]

In summary, in relation to age, sex, marital status, and living circumstances, there was little to distinguish the users of SSD day centres from those attending AHA day hospitals. Most users attending either type of unit described themselves as having a mental or emotional disorder. The users of day centres were more likely to name psychotic conditions, while more AHA users called their disorder 'depression'. Both of these groups were outnumbered by users who gave only the symptoms of their disorder, such as 'nerves' or 'withdrawal'. Although coming to a day unit is often a new experience for users, half to three-quarters had already lived for a time in psychiatric hospital. Once in day services, users seem to have a nearly even chance of staying over a year, but for the group who have attended less than a

[4] The information on discharges showed that the largest group of day centre and day hospital ex-users (30–33 per cent) took jobs in open employment, and that day hospital users did not transfer to day centres after leaving, since on average only 2 per cent of those discharged went on to day centres.

year discharge is more likely to occur if they are in day hospitals rather than day centres. All this information adds to a picture of more of those with chronic psychiatric disability attending day centres, although this should not be over-stressed as there appeared to be considerable overlap between the populations of the two sectors.

Who are the heads and staff?

Heads and staff may work in day units on either a full-time or part-time (sessional) basis, and the equivalent of about 3000 full-time paid workers come into direct contact with users every week in day units for the mentally ill in England and Wales. This number does not include the 1600 support staff, such as secretaries, domestics, and drivers, who back up the work of the other paid staff, nor does it include the 1000 or more volunteers who work part-time in day units on an unpaid basis. But the fact is that the paid staff are not equally distributed between SSD day centres and AHA day hospitals. Differences exist both in the absolute numbers of staff employed and in the training and qualifications which staff bring to the job.

If one assumed there were no differences between day hospitals and day centres, one might expect about three-quarters of all staff to be employed in AHA day hospitals while about a fifth might work in SSD day centres. However, the survey indicated some differences between the users of the two sectors. As many as half the SSD users were chronically disabled, following lengthy stays in psychiatric hospital, while the other half seemed to have more acute conditions. The majority of AHA users (about four-fifths) had more acute conditions, leaving a smaller chronic group of about a fifth. The actual distribution of employees in day services for the mentally ill showed that nine out of ten paid staff worked in AHA day hospitals. These wide differences in the number of staff working in the two sectors might be due simply to the proportions of acute and chronic users, but there is considerable overlap between the two populations, and an alternative assumption is that chronic users require more intensive attention if they are to progress. The qualifications of staff show further contrasts between the two sectors.

The equivalent of forty full-time doctors (including consultants and senior registrars) were employed by the AHA to work in the day hospitals in the survey. No doctors were seconded to or otherwise employed in the SSD day centres in the study, but in one day centre a psychiatrist did visit at least once a month. The equivalent of 74 full-time staff in the day hospitals held a psychiatric nursing qualification (RMN), while only two day centre workers were similarly qualified. Table 3.1 shows the distribution of these and other qualifications in more detail.

Table 3.1 Qualifications held by 'staff' in day units for the mentally ill[5]

Qualification	SSD 'Staff' (in 8 day centres ave. 33 places each)		AHA 'Staff' (in 29 day hospitals[6] ave. 40 places each)	
	No. of 'staff'	'Staff': User ratio	No. of 'staff'	'Staff': User ratio
Qualified Doctor	0	—	40	1:29
Registered Psychiatric Nurse (RMN) (including SRN plus RMN nurses)	2	1:132	74	1:16
Other nursing qualifications:				
State Registered Nurse (SRN)	1	1:264	36	1:36
State Enrolled Nurse (SEN)	1	1:264	31	1:37
Nursery Nurse (NNEB)	1	1:264	6	1:193
Occupational Therapy Diploma	2.5	1:106	29	1:40
Psychologist qualification	1	1:264	11	1:105
Social work qualification	0	—	8	1:145
Other university degree	2	1:132	5	1:232
Art or Art Therapy Diploma	1	1:264	2	1:580
Teacher's Certificate	2	1:132	0	—
Other qualifications	2	1:132	22	1:53
No qualification	9	1:29	29	1:40
Trade apprenticeship or vocational training	3	1:88	3	1:387
Student on placement	0	—	22	1:53
(No information)	4		13	
All 'staff'	31.5	1:8	331	1:3.5

[5] 'Staff' includes both heads and staff expressed in full-time equivalents, estimated from the interview sample. (Support staff are not included.) About 10 per cent of SSD and 20 per cent of AHA 'staff' held more than one qualification; such people appear under each qualification held.

[6] No information was received from two day hospitals.

How do people enter day services?

The entrance of users into day units

There were significant differences between how the largest groups of users in both sectors found their way into day services, even though nine out of ten users in both AHA and SSD units had been referred to the unit by a professional worker. Among day hospital users, this was most likely to have been a hospital doctor such as a consultant or registrar, but a third were referred by their family doctor. In contrast, among SSD users, social workers referred the most users to the centres. The only significant rival to this largely professional referral system came in the voluntary sponsored units, where about half the users had referred themselves, or first attended on the recommendation of a friend or family member.

The method of introduction to the day unit by the referring professional varied considerably. Few units had any scheme for informing potential users about the services that were offered. None of the day units had arranged for a member of staff to visit new users at home, and only two invited new users to visit the unit in advance of attendance. Since most units open at least five or six hours a day, and since most SSD users attend five days a week and AHA users attend only somewhat less frequently (just over a third attended five days a week), day services occupy a considerable portion of their days. The long periods some users will remain in day care has already been described. With this magnitude of time commitment from users, a full discussion of the possibilities and problems of day unit attendance, and perhaps contact with the unit in advance, may be of benefit to some.

Why heads and staff work in day units

Over three-quarters of heads and staff in day hospitals and two-thirds of their colleagues in day centres said they came to work in day services because the conditions were agreeable—the hours were good, there was no weekend or evening shift work, etc. Half as many in both sectors implied they came for more idealistic reasons: for example, a commitment to mental health work and in particular to services based in the community. For some staff members, these reasons coincided. A staff nurse indicated: 'I moved into the area and wanted to work in the community rather than the wards. I am divorced, so the hours suit my children.'

In common with many users, the bulk of staff have been associated with the day unit for long periods. The average length of service in day hospitals and centres was well over two years, and a fifth had been employed for over five years.

How do the people in day units spend their time?

The activities of users

Users were asked what they had expected to happen in the day unit when they first came. The largest group in SSD day centres, who could remember their expectations, said they thought they would work. The largest group in the day hospitals said that they expected to receive some form of treatment from a doctor, nurse, or therapist. Their expectations seemed to be borne out by the activities which were offered, but it was not possible to check if their recollections were correct.

Nearly all the day units for the mentally ill in the survey had a written programme of activities prepared for their units. Most offered a number of different activities each week, and sometimes each day, and each activity might represent a variety of tasks. That said, there was a marked similarity between the programmes of activities available in AHA day hospitals and SSD day centres.

Heads described the planned activities their day units offered under six headings. These are listed in order below, with the activity which was offered by the greatest number of day units for the mentally ill coming first. Following each activity, the three most frequently available tasks in both SSD and AHA day units are listed, with an indication of any differences between them:

1. *Social programme*: record sessions, table tennis, card games.

2. *Physical treatments*: by a doctor, nurse, or therapist—relaxation classes, special nursing care (injections or dressings, for example), medication dispensed by staff (AHA day hospitals) or keep fit classes (SSD day centres).

3. *Arts and Crafts*: sewing, painting, toymaking.

4. *Education Classes*: cookery, shopping activities, hair-dressing or make-up classes (AHA day hospitals) or drama classes (SSD day centres).

5. *Meetings*: therapy groups with a trained leader to discuss personal problems, discussion groups to discuss other matters related to the users, community meetings open to all to discuss the business of the day unit.

6. *Work, industrial or domestic*: work without tools (e.g. packing, sorting, labelling), work with non-powered hand tools (e.g. with staplers, hammers, needles), domestic work (e.g. cleaning, sweeping).

Figure 3.1 shows the proportion of SSD day centres and AHA day hospitals said to offer each activity in the week before the survey.

Users were also asked to describe what they did in the week before interview, and their replies added items to the list of activities. For

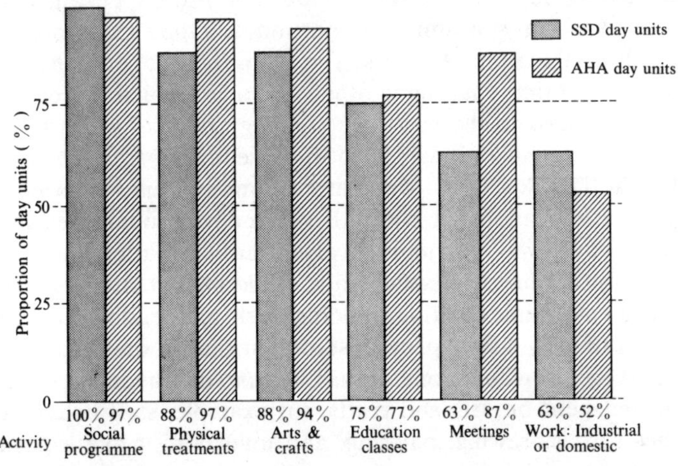

Fig. 3.1. Activities offered in day units.
(Information compiled from the heads of 8 SSD and 31 AHA units.)

example, the activity mentioned most often by users in both SSD and AHA day units was spending some time chatting to others. After chatting to others, the second most frequently mentioned activity among SSD users was arts and crafts. Although arts and crafts were available in most day units, they were taken up by three out of four SSD users compared to four out of seven AHA users. The second most frequently mentioned activity of AHA users was participating in meetings. About a quarter more day hospital than day centres included meetings or discussion groups in their programmes, but fewer users in both AHA and SSD units said they participated than might be expected, given the number of units offering meetings. About six out of ten users in SSD day centres where meetings or groups were offered, and seven out of ten in day hospitals, said they joined in.[7]

[7] In the case of meetings, this less than complete attendance was not accounted for by the user being away from the unit when the meetings were held, since only a few had been absent. Nor was it because the user was following a programme of activity designed for him or her which did not include meetings, since only a few units provided users with such individual programmes. And it was not because users were specially allocated to a member of staff, since the units where such a system operated were often those where a high proportion of users said they attended meetings and groups anyway. The fact that up to a third of users were not attending the available meetings may in some cases indicate that users are missing a benefit from the unit, and in others that users felt they got nothing out of meetings.

Users also described how they spent the greatest portion of their week. In SSD day centres, while about two-fifths spent most time doing arts and crafts, a similar proportion said they spent most time doing industrial or domestic work. The rest were split between a group that spent most time chatting to others and a group that was occupied doing chores around the unit (like running errands for the staff, or helping lay and clear away tables) most of the time. Only one SSD user spent most time during the week at meetings, and no one spent the most time at educational activities. In AHA day hospitals the concentration of activity was even more diverse. About a quarter of users said they spent most time on arts and crafts, while smaller groups said they spent either most time chatting, or doing work, or attending meetings.

In the staff view, users spent most of their time in ways that closely paralleled the users' opinions. It may be that, in scheduling so much time to be spent on arts and crafts, for example, staff believe that activities such as sewing, painting, and toymaking make a positive contribution to the well-being of users. Or it may be that the activities offered are all that are practicable, given the resources and time available, or the present state of knowledge about what might be beneficial to users. Towards the end of the chapter, users' perceptions of the benefits of attending existing day services will be discussed.

Heads' and staff's perceptions of their activities

The activities which heads and staff reported doing each week fell into eight broad categories. The issue was what definitions those working in units gave to the way they spent their time. The four most common definitions of activities in units for the mentally ill were:

1. *Administration*: including paperwork of any kind, answering the telephone, dealing with official visitors, sorting out transport problems, and so on.

2. *Exercising special professional skills*: including physiotherapy, occupational therapy, speech therapy, or other professional skill in individual or group sessions. It was up to the staff member to define whether, say, running a group was a special professional skill or one of the other activities.

3. *Social care activities*: could include taking part in community or group meetings, promoting educational activities, handling leisure or art materials by showing users how to do something, playing games with users, eating with users, and so on.

4. *Personal care*: including individual talks with users lasting longer

than ten minutes, consoling a user about anything, discussion of problems with a user's family, etc.

Other activities were defined around supervisory or domestic activities, or involved the physical care of users, or miscellaneous time spent having tea, resting, and so on.

The heads' week

More SSD and AHA heads spent the largest portion of their time doing administration than any other activity. On average, they spent a day and a half per week on administration: that is, about a third of the total hours they worked in the day unit. This time was roughly constant for all heads even though the AHA heads had somewhat more backup available from support staff such as administrators and secretaries than their SSD colleagues. So the actual position of 'head' of a day unit seemed to be the most influential factor in how people in that position described spending most of their time.

Apart from administration there were differences between heads in the two sectors. Nearly all the SSD heads said they divided another third of their working week between personal care and social care activities. But over half the AHA heads said they opted out of social care activities altogether, and a third said they did not involve themselves in personal care activities. However, those AHA heads who did undertake personal care activities spent a good deal of time on them—on average about a day and a half each week, which was nearly twice the time spent by equivalent SSD heads.[8]

The staff's week

The three largest staff groups in day hospitals—the nurses, doctors, and occupational therapists—all defined a major portion of their week as exercising their 'special professional skills', but there were also some differences between the groups. The qualified nurses and occupational therapists among the SSD workers on the whole attached similar definitions to their work as their AHA colleagues, so these definitions were not dependent on the sector in which staff members worked.

The largest staff group in day hospitals was the nurses. Registered psychiatric nurses (including those who were also state registered nurses) were the biggest group, comprising half the nurses. They were followed by the state registered nurses (25 per cent) and the state

[8] Three out of four AHA heads interviewed were registered psychiatric nurses and nearly all the rest were state registered nurses. Three out of seven SSD heads were also state registered nurses.

enrolled nurses (21 per cent). However, the specific qualifications which the nurses held did not seem to affect the pattern of activities they said occupied most of their time during the week. More nurses of every qualification said that most of their week was spent exercising what they defined as their nursing skills rather than in other activities. In contrast, the smallest group defined their most time-consuming task as personal care through individual talks with users,[9] and over half did not mention this activity at all. This was as true for registered psychiatric nurses as it was for those holding other nursing qualifications. What is not clear is whether those who defined the bulk of their time as 'special professional skills' included talking to patients as part of this.

Another large staff group in day hospitals—the trained occupational therapists—were even more likely than the nurses to consider the majority of their work time as using professional skills. Nearly all of them said they spent most time during the week using occupational therapy skills in individual or group sessions. Over half of them never defined their task as personal care. Social care of users was also said to occupy a relatively small proportion of the average occupational therapist's week (about a seventh, or less than a day a week, for a full-time therapist). Once again, talking to users, and undertaking their social care, is apparently seen by the occupational therapists as a professional skill rather than a matter of personal care.

The doctors in day hospitals presented a different picture. Although two-thirds placed some of their work into the category of exercising professional skills as doctors, the largest group defined the major proportion of their work in terms of the personal care they could offer to users. All doctors said they were involved in personal care, but whether or not this followed a particular approach was not specified. So in day hospitals where all three of the large staff groups had their own qualification base and their own brand of professional skills, the nurses and occupational therapists tended to define the majority of their work in terms of these skills first, while the doctors said they looked first to the personal care of users.[10]

---

[9] Talking to a member of staff about a personal problem was an opportunity afforded by the unit which over half the users in both AHA and SSD units said they had recently used.

[10] The more ambiguous position of many health workers including nurses and occupational therapists about their status as professionals may account for some of these differences. It may take a well-established and secure professional group like doctors to agree that talking to patients is not a professional skill. On the other hand, because many of the doctors interviewed were of pre-consultant status, they may not yet have been trained in how to regard talking to patients as a 'special professional skill'.

All the untrained staff in both sectors reported that personal care of users occupied the smallest portion of their week, but apart from that, the unqualified staff fell into three groups. The first group, in both day hospitals and day centres, simply defined the major use of their time along the lines of their job titles. Hence the cleaners said they spent most of their time on cleaning or other domestic activities and the secretarial staff said they spent most of their time on clerical or administrative tasks. But the second group (primarily in day hospitals) seemed to mirror the way the qualified staff to whom they worked spent their time. So, for instance, an untrained occupational therapy aide described spending the majority of her time exercising her 'special professional skills', and this happened similarly in the case of two untrained auxiliary nurses. The third group worked in day centres, where there were fewer trained staff to provide models. Most frequently this group defined their work as supervising users.

No simple link existed between the way heads and other staff defined the major use of their time and what they considered to be the most important aspect of their jobs. But about one task there was consensus. Three-fifths in SSD day centres, and two-fifths in AHA day hospitals, agreed that their most important task was to form relationships with users.[11] Some stressed particular facets of this when they mentioned the importance of talking to users and listening to them. One young nurse put it succinctly: 'The most important thing is to build up a relationship and rapport with patients, because without that you won't achieve anything.'

How heads and staff define the use of their time is, of course, complex: exercising professional skills, social care of users, personal care of users, administration etc., can be interpreted differently by different people. One man's 'personal care' may be another man's 'professional skill', and these definitions may in part depend on the importance placed on particular skills when obtaining a given qualification. How practical these differences in definitions are for the users and the heads and staff themselves is an open question which needs further exploration.

Users' judgements of the day units

What users said the day unit had done for them was considered in two parts. First, what particular aspects of their lives were affected by the

---

[11] Four-fifths of the staff in voluntary centres also agreed with their SSD and AHA colleagues about the importance of forming relationships with users.

unit, and second, what was the overall 'impact' of coming to the day unit? Again, few differences existed between users in SSD and AHA units concerning the particular aspects of their lives affected by day services, but there were differences in the second matter, the evaluations made of the overall 'impact' of the service on their lives.

First, taking the detailed descriptions of what aspects of their lives had been affected by day services, two aspects of life within the unit featured most frequently: how the user felt as an individual, and how the user functioned with other people in the unit. Where the user's personal feelings had been affected, he mentioned qualities in himself like confidence, concentration, morale, or happiness. Where his dealings with others in the unit had been affected, he mentioned social contacts, relationships with other users, or friendliness. Over a third of both day centre and day hospital users stated that their lives had been affected in both these ways. A thirty-year-old man who said he suffered from depression thought coming to the day hospital had '. . . cheered me up a bit. I think I've come out of my shell. I get things off my chest a bit by having someone to talk to.'

A third aspect of living upon which users commented was that day care simply provided them with somewhere to go to occupy their time during the day. A fifth of day hospital attenders and slightly more SSD users stated this: 'It gets me up in the morning, and occupies my time, but nothing else,' explained a young man in his twenties.

Only about one user in twenty—regardless of type of day unit —mentioned that the day unit had affected any of the following matters concerning their life outside the unit. First, there was the question of their ability to cope with social situations outside the day unit—e.g. 'I'm more considerate of other people and do more for my parents.' Second, there was their ability to perform new skills of the type one might learn at an adult education class—e.g. 'They have helped me to learn new words and they talk to me regularly so I can practise.' Third, there was the issue of their ability to take on new roles or revive old ones (for example, as father, wife, worker, or friend). Since it is precisely in areas such as these that people who are suffering from self-perceived mental disorders might be expected to have difficulties, it is perhaps surprising that so many users concentrated on describing their status within the day unit rather than on their lives away from the unit. This area needs more investigation, for as one man commented: 'The only snag is when you go away from the day hospital and go back home you're surrounded by things and people that were there when the trouble started.'

In evaluating the overall 'impact' of day unit attendance on users' lives, one of four judgements was made according to the user's predominant reaction:

1. If day unit attendance enabled the user to do some activity or if he thought he was now in a condition which was made possible by coming to the unit, *improvement* had taken place.

2. If day unit attendance had stopped, or in some way prevented, an event or condition which the user expected to adversely affect him, given his circumstances, *prevention* had taken place.

3. If day unit attendance kept the user going in personal, social, or physical ways, or simply provided occupation or a service (like meals), *maintenance* had taken place.

4. Where a user said day unit attendance had done nothing for him, or he made other negative comments related to this, the overall 'impact' was rated as *negative comments.*'

Some examples from the users' own descriptions of what coming to the day unit had done for them will help clarify these categories.

Improvement

It's made me much better in my health. I used to keep falling asleep all day long: it's woken me up. (A man in his mid-forties, who said he was suffering from schizophrenia—SSD day centre.)

The day unit has made me feel much calmer. I seem much more at ease now. It's taught me patience to think things out logically and clearly. (A young woman of 27 who stated she had always had a nervous disability—AHA day hospital.)

Prevention

It's helped me a lot. I'm a person who likes people and mixing with people. I'd hate just my own company. If this place shut down I would land up in hospital. (A 65-year-old lady who said she had a mental disorder and depression—SSD day centre.)

It's helped me a lot. I would have done something desperate when I lost my husband, but now I'm not so fed up. (A lady in her seventies who called her condition depression and said she had lost the use of her hand when her husband died—AHA day hospital.)

Maintenance

I meet people here. I don't think it's done anything else, I just like to talk. (A young woman in her early twenties who said she was schizophrenic—AHA day hospital.)

I can concentrate here and it occupies my time. (A 43-year-old women who was epileptic—SSD day centre.)

Negative comments

Coming here has done nothing for me. (A 58-year-old man who mentioned various physical complaints like a speech impediment following a stroke—SSD day centre.)

It's done nothing for me really, only I worry about what will happen in winter, not having a conveyance to the door. At short notice I couldn't tell you what it's done for me—I'm no different. (A man in his sixties, who recently had a mental breakdown—AHA day hospital.)

The overall 'impact' made by day unit attendance on the lives of users in SSD and AHA units is shown in Fig. 3.2. There was an exact match between the proportion of users in both types of units who described improvement. The largest difference came in the proportion of users describing maintenance, with over half the AHA users but somewhat fewer SSD users experiencing it. About a quarter of all SSD users thought by coming to the day unit prevention had taken place, but here somewhat fewer AHA users had experienced this. However, the differences were not large enough to be statistically significant.

In the AHA day hospitals, the length of time users had attended the unit made little difference to their descriptions. Those who had been attending for different periods—six months, a year, two to five years, or five years or more—were distributed very similarly to all the users of day hospitals described below in Fig. 3.2. But in SSD day centres, while the proportion of users describing prevention stayed about the same for different periods of attendance, the proportion describing maintenance went down with longer attendance, and the proportion describing improvement went up. Negative comments were made only by users who had attended the day centre for two years or more. So in day centres, the proportion of users who described improvement

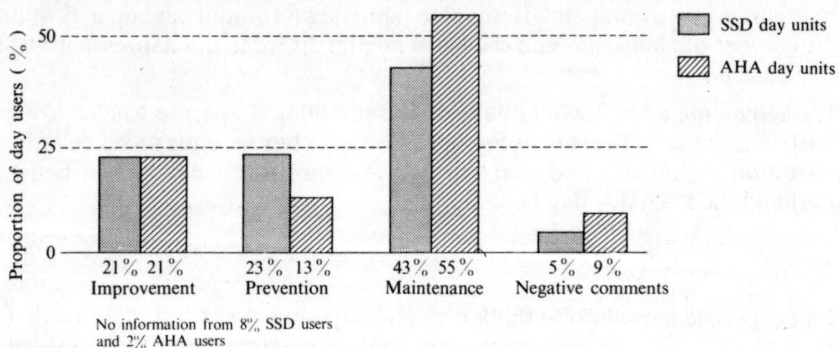

Fig. 3.2. 'Impact' of day unit attendance.
(Information compiled from 39 SSD and 126 AHA users.)

increased the longer they had attended, but at the same time as many as a fifth of the longer attenders began to make negative comments about the 'impact' of day services on their lives.[12]

Describing the reported 'impact' of day unit attendance on the lives of users in terms of improvement, maintenance, and prevention may be relevant to current users of day units as well as staff and others interested in day services, because it provides one method of assessing the strengths and weaknesses of continued attendance. If maintenance is intended as an appropriate outcome for a given user and the user accepts this, he or she may be receiving the maximum benefit possible from day unit attendance. But if a user hopes for improvement by attending a day unit, or that prevention of some unwanted condition might occur, a report of maintenance may indicate a gap in the service. Notably few negative comments about the impact of day services were made by users, but it is fair to comment that users who were very dissatisfied may already have stopped attending.[13]

Discussion

This chapter has outlined the day services provided by area health authorities and social services departments which exist to assist mentally ill people in England and Wales. As already mentioned, the government White Paper (1975) endorsed the separation of day services into two sectors: AHA day hospitals were to have an acute treatment bias, while SSD day centres were to have a primary commitment to social care. The rationale was that establishing day hospitals would encourage people to seek treatment earlier, thus preventing more serious episodes and possible in-patient admission. There was also an implicit belief that in-patients could be discharged earlier to day hospitals and it was thought that higher levels of staffing would make it possible to provide a better service. On the other hand, the day centres were to plan to meet the immediate social rather than medical

[12] Users' feelings of depression in the past month did not appear to affect the overall 'impact' of day unit attendance which they described. The largest group of users, from those who said they had not felt depressed to those whose description of depression was rated as 'considerable', said they had experienced maintenance in the day unit. The smallest group, with one exception, made negative comments.

[13] The question of what credence can be given to users' views as compared to independent professional opinions is controversial in social research. This study has supported the assumption that the user's view of his own personal reality is more valid than independent views. This runs counter to the assumption that a professional judgement is more 'objective' evidence than the user's view of himself. A separate but related issue is the interviewing method by which the users' views were obtained; details of this are given in the final reports of the survey.

needs of their users. Each individual's present level of functioning was to be assessed and a programme of activities designed to help him reach better adjustment. It was accepted that some users would be discharged from day centres, but the need of some for long-term shelter was implicit. Thus one measure of this policy is whether each sector provides a distinctive package for the people using each service.

It is quite clear that the heads and staff interviewed had absorbed at least some of the distinctive aims outlined by the White Paper. More of those working in the AHA sector said their units aimed to offer clinical assessment and treatment, while more SSD workers said their day centres aimed to provide a range of concrete practical services to users. But apart from these different aims, there was much common ground. In both sectors, roughly equal proportions said their units aimed to keep people out of hospitals, and there was also agreement about trying to return users to independent living in the community. It could be argued that these similarities of aims run counter to the intention of the White Paper which emphasized the distinctiveness of the two sectors at the expense of what they shared. Further similarities were seen, for example, in the way staff in the two sectors defined the use of their time, and for that matter in how users used their time too, since the activities offered in both sectors were so alike. The most striking staff difference related to the numerous clinically trained staff (e.g. doctors, nurses, and occupational therapists) employed in day hospitals, which probably gave a boost to the achievement of the clinical assessment and treatment aim.

Amongst the users more similarities than differences emerged, too. The main difference was that acute users (conservatively defined as those with no previous stay, or a stay of less than a year, in psychiatric hospitals) did not all attend AHA day hospitals, since the survey showed that about half the SSD users were also acute. While it is true that SSD day centres had more chronic users than AHA day hospitals, there was a wider area of similarity between users of the two sectors than might be expected by taking the recommendations of the White Paper literally.

A number of factors may account for this apparent overlap. The first is the method of the national survey itself. A national survey aggregates the views and characteristics of people in a wide cross-section of day units, and thus disguises a great deal of variation between individual units and authorities. Therefore, it is wrong to suppose that a national pattern of staffing or user views can predict the way individual day centres or day hospitals will operate. For example, how closely day centres and day hospitals are situated to each other might influence their operation and help determine the extent of overlap. In fact only six of the thirteen authorities surveyed had both AHA and SSD day units (including just one of the five counties), and on the whole the day hospitals in these authorities where there was also a day centre were not more specialized and could not be distinguished from the rest. That is, overall, their aims were similar to those day hospitals in authorities without day centres; the proportion of long-term users attending them was similar to those without day centres, and they did not discharge significantly more users. Nor when discharged did it appear that any more of their users transferred to the day centre. So the general implication is that day hospitals and day centres run quite independently even when they are in the same area. The exception to this was one outer-London authority, with both day hospitals and day centres, where there was a carefully planned administrative pathway of care between the two sectors. The day hospitals in this authority discharged twice the national average number of users, and three times the national average went on to the local SSD day centre. But this kind of individual difference was rare enough not to influence the national aggregate.

In addition, the apparent overlap between the AHA and SSD sectors may be accounted for by certain social and organizational developments. Over the past decade the health sector has shown an increasing interest in extending the hospital into the community. The day hospitals themselves illustrate this, but there are other extensions being developed—not without controversy. For instance, who is best to follow up users after leaving day hospitals—social workers, or the new community psychiatric nurses? There were very few community psychiatric nurses working from a day hospital base. However, four out of five day hospitals in the survey referred some patients to a community psychiatric nurse for follow-up. Their presence points to a possible health-sector trend towards maintaining a self-contained follow-up service which obviates the need for referral to social services. Alongside this, psychiatrists seem to have become more interested in extending their work to deal with the challenging field of the secondary handicaps of chronic patients, thus complicating the precept that the AHA is the acute treatment sector.

One or two of the day hospitals were interested in dealing with mental illness outside the medical context of the clinical model, and had adopted some of the features of the 'therapeutic community'. However, these day hospitals remained under medical direction. In a few SSD day centres there was a trend towards the view that mental illness could be helped outside a medical context altogether. This was the view of two SSD day centres in an inner-London borough, and this model also had been adopted by a number of day units for other user groups such as ex-offenders and young families. In fact many of the young parents in the national survey attending family day centres were rated as depressed as those users in units for the mentally ill who have been discussed already. It is worth noting that people labclled as 'mentally ill' may attend other day facilities too, such as sheltered workshops and day units catering for more than one user group; for example, the physically handicapped and the mentally ill.

The fact that both sectors provided similar services in a largely independent way was reinforced by the fact that the majority of referrals were being made along congruent paths—SSD social workers referred the most users to SSD day centres, and hospital doctors referred the most users to AHA day hospitals. On the other hand, the voluntary centres accepted self-referrals, uncommon in both the other sectors. However, at least one new centre in London, jointly funded by voluntary and statutory agencies, has adopted the self-referral system and will extend the idea of users helping each other with their difficulties. These are further developments in the trend towards treating mental illness outside a medical context.

Achieving a path for users out of day units is a goal shared by some staff in both the AHA and SSD sectors. On discharge figures alone, this goal appears to be achieved more frequently in day hospitals, but discharge is not the same as resettlement in the community. Only about a third of the users of both SSD and AHA sectors considered that any staff member in the unit had discussed their future with them. So although day hospitals discharge more quickly, the majority of users appear not to be prepared systematically for this change.

Clearly, providing for the range of requirements of those suffering varying degrees of mental illness at all stages is an enormous task. Whether the present differences between the services of AHA day hospitals and SSD day centres are distinct enough to offer real options to users and those trying to assist them is debatable, and needs further investigation. On the other hand, it is also important to consider how desirable it would be to perfect the distinctions set out in the current White Paper, and what repercussions this would have on staff and users. Other experience has shown that creating a venue for chronic care may depress staff and undermine user progress.

The dilemma of separate day services may be resolved with the help of the users themselves. Although government policy explicitly encourages users to take part in planning and organizing day services, this kind of participation was found to occur very little in practice. The more users are encouraged to help shape their own services, the more the relevance of separate services will be tested.

FURTHER READING

Bennett, D. H. (1976). Day treatment in England. In *Adult psychiatric day treatment proceedings*. Paper given at the First Multi-disciplinary National Forum on Adult Psychiatric Day Treatment. (Available from University of Minnesota, 206 Nolte Centre, 315 Pillsbury Drive S.E., Minneapolis, Minnesota.)

Cross, K. W., Hassall, C. and Gath, D. (1972). Psychiatric day-care, the new chronic population?, *Br. J. Prev. Soc. Med.*, **26**, 199–204.

DHSS (1975). *Better services for the mentally ill*. Cmnd 6233. HMSO, London.

National Day Care Project (1978). *Adult day care: selected reading*. National Institute for Social Work, 5/7 Tavistock Place, London WC1.

Wing, J. K. and Hailey, A. M. (1972). *Evaluating a community psychiatric service: the Camberwell register 1964–71*, Oxford University Press.

4 Residential care for the mentally disabled

Peter Ryan

The acid test of a community service lies in whether it can meet the needs of those people with severe mental disabilities who, in former times, would have become long-stay patients in psychiatric hospitals. Because of improvements in treatment many, of course, no longer become seriously disabled. Some do not even need to be admitted to hospital at all. Nevertheless, there is good evidence that a substantial group of people still do need residential and day care or shelter (see Chapter 1). An effective service must be able to cope with their needs without giving rise to intolerable burdens on families or on the community at large and without allowing a drift into destitution.

This chapter is concerned with the principles of residential care for the 'adult mentally ill' who do not need to be in hospital but, for a variety of reasons, are unable to live at home or maintain themselves in their own accommodation. The term 'care' includes the provision of sheltered or subsidized accommodation for people who do not need any other kind of rehabilitation or treatment.

There is general agreement that the number of places available has not kept pace with the need created by the steady movement, during the past twenty-five years, away from using psychiatric hospitals to meet mainly social needs. The government White Paper, *Better services for the mentally ill*, admitted, in 1975, that 'by and large the nonhospital community resources are still minimal . . . The failure, for which central government is as much at fault as local government, to develop anything approaching adequate services is perhaps the greatest disappointment of the last 15 years.' The guidelines laid down were for 4–6 places per 100000 population in short-stay hostels and 15–24 places per 100000 in long-stay accommodation.

Even counting the places provided by voluntary and private organizations registered with local authorities, only 43 per cent of the minimum recommended places were available in 1975. In 1973–4, £15 million was spent on personal social services for the mentally ill, of which less than half was for residential and day care facilities. The expenditure on residential care for the mentally ill accounted for only 0.04 per cent of local authority expenditure in 1974–5.

It seems unlikely that there will be a major increase in the amount spent on the mental health services in the near future and it is all the more important, therefore, to consider not only the numbers of residential places needed, but also the extent to which they can be provided more economically while still meeting need. Three types of function have traditionally been provided for in hospitals that could theoretically be carried out in alternative accommodation outside. (The group needing long-term 'hospital' care is discussed in Chapter 1.)

First, there are homeless people who are not severely disabled except in the sense that they are unable to compete for housing on the open market; because of poverty, incapacity for employment, and the lack of motivation common in some psychiatric disorders such as schizophrenia. Group homes or other subsidized housing schemes, set up by housing associations and paid for through grants and social security payments enable this group to live relatively normal lives, since they are able to look after themselves and their homes, do the shopping and pay the rent with minimal supervision. Some of the 'old long-stay' at present living in unstaffed villas or wards in psychiatric hospitals (and possibly some of those in supervised hostels) can make use of this kind of provision.

Second, there is a somewhat more disabled group of people who find it difficult to carry out all the domestic activities necessary to maintain themselves and their home and who need a degree of care as well as financial support. This is the group looked after in the hostels of the Mental After-Care Association and, more recently, in other voluntary and statutory sheltered accommodation. It is not expected that they will be 'resettled' elsewhere but that the hostel is their permanent home. The degree of supervision required varies. Some hostels require a high staff–resident ratio, with well-trained staff available; others require minimal supervision.

Third, there is a group of people who are thought to need 'rehabilitation' in order to prepare them for independent living. 'Half-way houses' have been set up in order to facilitate the transition between hospital and community, with the intention that residents will be working within a few months of admission and can thus move on to their own accommodation. This third kind of hostel was prominent in the plans of voluntary bodies and local authorities during the 1950s and 1960s and still seems to dominate the plans of some authorities today. D. H. Clark and L. W. Cooper described one of the first transitional hostels in 1960. Two related problems had become apparent. One was that it was difficult to find sufficient hospital patients who fitted the fairly strict selection criteria. Most people who had the potential to find work within a few months preferred to leave hospital at once. This led to under-occupancy. The other problem was that even those who were selected had great difficulty in moving on when their period in the hostel was theoretically over. This led to a feeling of failure, both among residents and among staff.

In spite of this prescient paper most hostels set up by local authorities during the 1960s had the avowed intention to provide for the transition from hospital to community. A series of further studies by J. C. Fletcher, G. H. Mountney, and E. Durkin called attention to the management problems of these hostels. Mountney warned that half-way houses could become 'almost a replica of the worst aspects of old institution life but at almost twice the cost'.

A national postal survey by R. Z. Apte, published in 1968, suggested that a large number of hostels were restrictive in their practices and concluded, 'without a clarification of purpose, the half-way house could turn into a diffuse and aimless institution, similar to the *workhouse* of former years'. Apte thought that hostels that provided permissive environments were likely to have higher discharge rates. 'A permissive atmosphere encourages the resident's ego to return to more autonomous functioning and promotes meaningful solid interaction with other individuals. Through the maintaining of high responsibility expectations, it fosters the re-establishment of the resident into more socially adaptive and gratifying roles.'

A further, and much more detailed study of hostels was made in 1973 by Sheila Hewett and the present author. People aged 16–65 who were supported financially, by three south-London boroughs, in residential accommodation for the 'adult mentally ill', were interviewed, as were members of staff. Apart from one small housing association all the residents were living in hostels. One of these (run by the local authority) was within the area but most (run by voluntary associations) were not. Several were situated in coastal towns a long way from London.

In contrast to Apte's conclusion, we found that all the hostels studied provided 'permissive' environments. Moreover, there was no evidence that hostels intended to be short-stay were more permissive than those intended as permanent homes. If anything, a greater emphasis on 'rehabilitation' required a greater degree of structure and therefore of limitation on the lives of residents. Only nine 'restrictive' practices were described in more than half of the hostels visited. Many of these were quite reasonable, in the sense that they would be acceptable in most normal households; knowing where residents were at weekends, who would be in for meals, not having a choice of main dishes at mealtimes, not smoking in bedrooms because of fire regulations, and being called in the morning in order to get to work.

On the other hand, restrictions on visitors (who usually had to leave by 11pm) might occasionally have been irksome. Medication was usually handed out by wardens rather than being left to the responsibility of residents. Perhaps less defensibly, staff sometimes entered residents' rooms without knocking. There was also a general tendency for residents to be called by their christian names while staff were given their titles. Compared with an ordinary family environment, however, these hostels could not be called restrictive.

A further survey was carried out by the author in 1976 in order to compare management practices and characteristics of residents and staff in a range of non-hospital residential settings. Their place in the overall scheme of services was also investigated. Four hostels and three networks of group homes, situated in four north London boroughs, were chosen for study because, between them, they were thought to provide as good a service as existed anywhere in the country and to incorporate innovating features. One of the hostels, for example, was purpose-built for 20 residents, and was run on corporate management lines, with staff attempting to maximize resident participation. One of the local authority housing departments was closely involved in another scheme, providing two networks of group homes, one supervised by social workers, the other by community nurses from the local psychiatric hospital (where there was a group home preparation unit). Another scheme was centred on a large purpose-built hostel whose staff also provided supervision for a group home preparation unit, a self-care annex, and a small block of flats; overall supervision being provided by a community psychologist.

A more formal account of the results of this survey has been presented elsewhere (Ryan and Wing: see suggestions for further reading). The rest of this chapter is based mainly upon these results and on those obtained from the 1973 survey by Hewett and Ryan. The characteristics of short- and long-stay hostels, group homes, and family care are considered separately and attention is then given to the problems of ensuring that they are part of an overall service which is both comprehensive and integrated.

Short-stay hostels

Objectives

When the first 'half-way houses' were set up, it was assumed that large numbers of people in psychiatric hospitals needed rehabilitation in order to help them overcome the disabilities of institutionalism and that they would then be able to resume an independent life in society. It had been demonstrated that such help, given in hospital, did have useful results (see Chapter 1). The aim, therefore, was to resettle people within a relatively short space of time, say six months to a year. The term 'resettlement' meant supporting oneself independently by means of one's wages or salary.

This aim became broader and less precise during the subsequent decade. The staff of one of the hostels surveyed in 1976 (Hostel 2) expressed their 'corporate management' philosophy as follows, 'We're trying to create a community where people can have relations without becoming confused and depressed as many have been in more restrictive institutions such as mental hospitals', and 'We're helping to live an autonomous life in the community with as few restrictions as possible'. To a lesser degree, all the hostels in the 1976 survey expressed this kind of intention, but they still adhered also to the earlier aim of achieving independence for inmates, e.g.: 'The aims are to encourage each resident to achieve maximum independence with a view to a final placement in the community. This is achieved by residents progressing from the hostel to a bed-sitting room and then to a flat before they move back into the community when no longer in need of support.'

Selection of residents

The selection of residents is carried out in different ways according to the philosophy of rehabilitation adopted by hostel managers. Hostels where residents were encouraged to participate in management also gave them an opportunity to influence the selection of new residents.

Thus in one hostel, every applicant was visited at home or in hospital by a staff member and a resident. Those who passed this interview were invited to the hostel for a meal to meet other residents and staff. A consensus decision was made by a panel consisting (for example) of three staff members, two referring social workers, and six hostel residents. The criteria for selection included motivation to benefit from a short stay, ability to fit into the existing group of residents, and positive qualities that might be of value in the hostel. A balance was preserved between the sexes.

By contrast, in a 'low consultation' hostel, residents were only marginally involved in selection. Applicants were screened by the warden, and suitable candidates were then seen by a panel consisting of warden, psychiatric adviser and Area Social Service Officer. Only after passing this second screen was an applicant invited to spend a weekend at the hostel. The results of the two selection methods were not noticeably different. Both emphasized a lack of disturbed behaviour or active social withdrawal.

Characteristics of residents

In both surveys, it was clear that residents were 'single homeless persons', three-quarters of whom had never married while most of the rest were separated or divorced. Very few had had a lasting sexual relationship even at their best. There had been a long history of previous hospital residence; about one-third having been in hospital a total of five years or more.

There were some interesting differences between the two surveys. In 1973, 73 per cent had previously been given a diagnosis of schizophrenia compared with 43 per cent in 1976, the difference being made up by more residents with a previous diagnosis of personality disorder or neurosis. The proportion of males in the earlier survey was 50 per cent compared to 63 per cent in 1976. The proportions in the two surveys aged 45 and over were 60 per cent and 30 per cent. In 1973, 80 per cent of residents of short-stay hostels were working fulltime compared with only 14 per cent in 1976. In 1973, 35 per cent of residents had been in the hostels for less than one year (i.e. most were long-stay), whereas in 1976, 67 per cent had stayed for less than a year.

These differences might suggest that the group within the 'old long-stay' hospital population who could relatively easily be found work had already been discharged or were less often considered and that a more mixed group, including some 'new long-stay' were being admitted, but with much less chance of finding work. (The general unemployment rate had of course increased in the interim.) The hostels studied in 1976 had been set up relatively recently so that the difference in length of hostel residence cannot yet be evaluated.

The chief behavioural characteristic in both surveys was social withdrawal though this was not as severe as in the 'old long-stay' hospital populations described by Sheila Mann and Wendy Cree. In the 1976 survey, a majority (69 per cent) of residents said they did not want to leave the hostel. Further information about behaviour is given in the next section together with a description of the methods used to cope with problems.

Rehabilitation

Maximizing autonomy has been one of the central elements of the approach to rehabilitation adopted in the therapeutic communities set up in psychiatric hospitals and the staff of short-stay hostels have been powerfully influenced by it. Apte expressed the philosophy of 'permissive' environments as follows: 'A permissive atmosphere encourages the resident's ego to return to more autonomous functioning and promotes meaningful solid interaction with other individuals. Through the maintaining of high responsibility expectations, it fosters the re-establishment of the resident into more socially adaptive and gratifying roles.'

In the earlier study, many hospital staff, in practice, equated work with resettlement. Holding down a steady job was an index of success. In 1976, however, there were conflicting views. One group of staff argued that their task was not to 'push people out into dead-end jobs as factory fodder'. Residents who were employed nevertheless enjoyed their jobs and wanted to continue despite the low pay and manual work. Fewer than 10 per cent wanted more responsibility. The emphasis that hostel staff place on outside employment is probably the single most important factor determining the kind of life residents lead.

Hostels vary in the extent to which group meetings are used as a means of rehabilitation. Some place great emphasis on them, in the hope that residents will be able to talk about their problems at work and in relationships with others, thus learning to interact constructively and with less conflict. Other hostels place more emphasis on 'domestic therapy', with group meetings focused on problems of personal hygiene, saving money, shopping, and so on.

In the 1976 survey, a 'rehabilitation index' was used to describe the nature of the interventions used in hostels. Each member of staff was first asked which problems were presented by individual residents and which they thought required intervention. The commonest single problem was avoidance of social contact, and several other problem behaviours were probably part of the same syndrome: poor performance of chores, overdependence, underinvolvement, underassertion. Together, these accounted for half of all the problems mentioned. Others were overassertion, work difficulties, anxiety about leaving, inconsistency, low self-esteem, depression, and inappropriate social behaviour.

Some examples of social withdrawal and the way that staff tried to deal with it will be given in order to illustrate 'rehabilitation' in action. The following examples are taken from the hostel with the corporate management philosophy (Hostel 2) since staff there were particularly concerned to encourage participation. In most instances, withdrawal was seen as a severe incapacity to use social skills in initiating and maintaining relationships.

He worries us. He's the same with everybody. Two of us meet once a week to make regular contact and to try to initiate conversation with him. It's slow and heavy. You can't go very deep and you have to be very slow and patient.

Her relationship to the other residents is non-existent. People like her but she doesn't talk with anybody. She only really talks with staff. We do talk with her about her feelings of isolation and she tends to be closer with women. Some of the men here she really hates.

He comes into the office very freely. In the office he does attempt to make contact but outside in the dining room for example he just stares around silently.

He's overdependent on the hostel for its social contacts. He needs to have a supportive environment. He has resisted going outside. He wants to stay on here indefinitely.

In one of the hostels (Hostel 1) staff were unusually well-trained and made conscious use of various 'technical' skills such as contract bargaining, confrontation, desensitization, sensitivity groups, family therapy, and insight counselling. They held weekly budget planning groups (deciding e.g. the menu for the coming week) and a regular weekly house meeting. Every hostel member, staff and residents, cooked one evening meal per week. In addition two staff members met every two weeks with each resident to discuss progress. Nevertheless, half the interventions made in response to the problem behaviours they reported were non-technical in nature and in 17 per cent of instances no intervention was made at all.

She tends not to make contact with us unless something's very wrong. I'm frustrated in that I know she feels better when she does talk, yet you really have to dig it out of her. Often she just won't talk unless she's bursting. All I can do is let her know that I am always available.

She is very dependent. She likes us to help her to get up but we've discouraged this. We think she should be able to get up by herself. She'll take all the attention we can give her. She says she has to become dependent before she can become independent but we don't think this is true . . . We've got her to fill a graph of her mood swings every day so she can take a check on how different she feels. We discussed with her whether there's a regular pattern in her swings of mood.

In the other two hostels in the 1976 survey staff made use of 'technical' interventions even less although they described much the same problems. They responded with encouragement and support.

He is almost never spontaneous and then he comes to ask advice on practical questions. We try to reduce his anxiety by doing things with him, such as card games. There is not much you can do with him or for him. He has reached a plateau.

We've got to nail him down to stand any chance of persuading him to do his chores. We've got to get him to do it specifically while you're standing there watching him, otherwise he simply won't.

The environment as seen by residents

During the 1976 survey, residents were asked to comment on their experiences in hostels; particularly on how they got on together, on what life was like, and on how staff managed situations that arose from day to day. All such comments were recorded. They varied a good deal but the range was much the same in all hostels and in approximately the same proportions of positive, neutral, and negative. Examples of positive comments are given below, followed by examples of negative comments. It should be remembered that the most vocal are probably the least handicapped.

HOSTEL 1

We go out a lot together . . . We help new residents by making them feel welcome and at home and help them adjust.

Staff leave residents to clean their own rooms. If they did keep on at you, I would feel I was a child being nagged at by mother, whereas we're quite capable of doing things for ourselves.

If you just sit around doing nothing you think what use am I in life? but the nice thing about this place is that society outside is too big and scary, but this is my special place.

We tolerate people's peculiarities here. Here you're accepted, so we are very reluctant to let people leave for no good reason.

They [staff] try to sort out your problems for you. They take you as an individual.

HOSTEL 2

When I started here I was very shallow and withdrawn. Some people here have helped me out of that.

Staff show you how to prepare things. I've learnt most of my cooking from them at weekends.

Sometimes people here build up relationships or groups get together that trust each other a lot and quite a lot of different feelings get expressed.

Staff are very open with residents.

Residents are always consulted on important decisions.

With some staff I get on very well, because they are frank and open in their opinions. You get the impression they are just the same as you are. You don't get that in hospital.

HOSTEL 3

There is a very helpful spirit of sympathy and understanding.

I have been given quite a bit of personal assistance of a highly personal nature. For example, last week, staff gave me advice about how I should perm my hair.

We always go out in the evenings.

One of the residents cooked the meal tonight as the cook was off sick.

Residents always know where they are with staff. Staff are individuals and you get to know who you are dealing with.

If you've got anything to say to staff you can go to see them any time.

HOSTEL 4

Making friends here comes with time; the same with any other friendship.

There are no rows here; or any disagreements either.

I change my furniture any way I want.

The thing is, this place becomes a home for me round about dinnertime . . . At weekends, we have a way of cooperating to make sure that the food is prepared. It is done by mutual respect; just like being in a big family.

They [staff] try and make this place as much a home as possible. The last thing people want is to go back to mental hospital.

Staff will tell you if you are looking nice or if you have bought a new dress recently.

Staff are doing a job as well as trying to live here, whereas we are just trying to live.

The following are examples of negative comments.

HOSTEL 1

For some of us it's too easy here. There's too much support. You feel you can stay here forever.

I feel, 'My God, I'm not getting anywhere.' But you can't really tell them [staff] because it would hurt their feelings. It's that way altogether.

They talk about their problems all the time; you can't get away from it. I go out in the evenings sometimes to avoid the psychiatric atmosphere inside.

You feel like you're being watched all the time. It makes it kind of official somehow.

HOSTEL 2

There is a lot of mischief; vendettas even. I had the buttons slashed off my coat, my slippers went missing and the radio was turned on full blast when I was out of my room.

This place stinks. There is a useless pretence at conversation but you don't say what you feel.

Mostly you sit watching TV in silence. It is like being alone amongst a lot of people.

Staff are pretty confused themselves. There is a lot of confusion here. It would be better if the meetings were more open.

Staff don't control medication properly. We have had two suicides for that reason. One guy kept on making suicide attempts but nothing was done.

They leave people to stew without any help.

There are not enough staff here to do the more skilled things. They allow too much time for people to do nothing.

HOSTEL 3

Staff reckon I fit in here but I reckon I don't.

Some people go out but most just sit around.

We talk about staff behind their backs but shut up if they come along.

The group meetings don't get you anywhere.

People spend a lot of time in bed.

Unless you are going to work, staff don't bother a lot with you.

HOSTEL 4

It would be better if things were more organized by staff.

People like to sit down after dinner, watch TV, feel sorry for themselves, and talk about their illness.

Something more should be done for us to structure our time.

I think the staff are untidy themselves.

I still feel inferior to the staff.

The trouble here is that you are left to your own devices most of the time. People are hanging around here waiting for an organizer to come on the scene, but we can't all be organizers.

Evaluation

No strict evaluation of the effectiveness of rehabilitation procedures used in hostels, comparable to projects carried out in hospitals, has yet been undertaken, and claims must therefore be very limited. Neither the 1973 nor the 1976 surveys incorporated controls or a follow-up of discharged residents. Nevertheless, information was gathered which is relevant to an assessement of whether the aims of hostel management and staff were realistic.

These aims are twofold. In the first place, by definition, short-stay hostels offer only temporary accommodation and must therefore aim to help residents move to less dependent settings; at best, to paid work which will enable them to rent their own accommodation. In the 1973 survey, 80 per cent of 'short-stay' residents were indeed working but it was evident that most would not have been better off if they were discharged. Two-thirds had been resident for more than a year and thus were technically 'long-stay'.

In 1976, this position was reversed. Only a quarter of the residents were employed (including part-time work) but two-thirds had been resident in the hostels for less than a year (although 59 per cent wanted to stay). In part, this is due to a change of clientele. There were more younger men with personality disorders and neuroses who tended to stay for shorter periods of time. People with a past history of schizophrenia are less likely to be discharged and have more need for shelter, even when working. They react less favourably to group therapy. Such distinctions are, however, played down in hostel practice. Nevertheless, with the further growth of unemployment, and the recognition that much of it is likely to persist for at least a decade, these problems are likely to increase. Since there were few differences between hostels, in either study, in the extent to which residents were able to find employment, there is little evidence that a more or a less 'permissive' environment has much relevance to this aim.

The second type of aim is more limited; to improve the social functioning of residents and improve their quality of life. Again there was little evidence of difference between the hostels in spite of the fact that, in the 1976 survey, two (Hostels 1 and 2) utilized special methods ('technical' staff skills and 'corporate management') to achieve the aim. The author accepts, as a value judgement, that it is better to try to increase the participation and autonomy of residents, but it cannot yet be claimed that there is evidence that particular management techniques do achieve this.

One relevant type of evidence is the number of decisions taken by residents as compared with those taken by staff. In the 1976 survey, hostel residents reported that about a third of all decisions were taken solely on their own responsibility, while about a half were taken solely by staff. Hostels 3 and 4 allowed residents rather less responsibility than Hostels 1 and 2, mainly because fewer decisions were taken jointly. This result probably did stem from different staff attitudes.

Long-stay hostels

The first organization to provide after-care accommodation for the mentally ill (the Mental After-Care Association) explicitly recognized the needs of the long-stay patient, but this example has in most respects never been followed. However, the 1975 White Paper explicitly recognizes the need for long-stay accommodation, and gives priority in its planning recommendations to the provision of long-term care:

The housing needs of patients who have been in mental illness hospitals for many years but no longer require continuing medical and nursing care should not be overlooked. Obviously the rate at which such patients can return to the community will be constrained by the community's capacity to meet their underlying needs, both for housing and social support, but there should be an underlying recognition that hospital is not as satisfactory as home.

The Mental After-Care Association (MACA) was started by the Reverend Hawkins of Colney Hatch Hospital in 1879. Over the years it expanded as a result of the support it received, initially from patrons. The expansion, however, never went beyond London or the South East. At the end of 1976, it had eight long-stay hostels, housing 248 people. It is still the only organization that specializes in providing permanent hostel shelter.

Three long-stay MACA hostels were included in the 1973 survey, all located along the south-east coast. None of the residents interviewed, all of whom had previously lived in London before entering hospital, had the opportunity of re-establishing contact with their 'local' community. Only one of the three hostels housed both men and women. One of the hostels had previously been a hotel. The other two were large, terraced houses. Their rhythm of activity was very different from those of the short-stay hostels. It was most poignantly expressed by one of the wardens who said: 'We're growing old together; in ten years time this will be an old peoples' home.' Residents were not expected either to work or to attend a day-centre, although one or two had part-time seasonal jobs. Most of the residents lived a life that was to a great extent within the hostels themselves. Breakfast would be served (cooked by staff) at 8.30 a.m. and anyone who was late arriving would be 'hurried up' by staff. After breakfast, residents would spend the next two or three hours carrying out their allotted chores. (One lady was much attached to cleaning the toilet; although staff had frequently suggested a change, she would not hear of it.) This would be followed by mid-morning tea and biscuits, after which some residents (in the summer at least) would go for a walk along the sea front, and perhaps have a cup of tea in a cafe. After lunch, some would go for a walk, or go into town, perhaps to buy some stamps or post a letter. Others would prefer to sit down and rest. It was not at all unusual to see eight or ten residents resting in chairs along the sitting-room walls, much as they did in old-fashioned hospital wards.

Although short-stay rehabilitation aims (i.e. work and independent living) were beyond the capacity of nearly all the residents, staff nevertheless did try to help residents overcome unusual or withdrawn behaviour. One lady, for example, was always ten minutes late for every meal. The warden had tried all kinds of ploys (including making her alarm clock ten minutes fast) to help her become more punctual.

He had not succeeded. This illustrates perhaps the greatest difficulty that staff were faced with. For all these residents, the capacity to learn more adaptive patterns of behaviour was extremely limited. None of them would ever live independently or work at a fulltime job, and some would be likely to continue their odd or ritualistic behaviour. Some, however, might well change in small but significant ways, and it was with these residents that staff experienced their greatest reward. One lady, for example, had initially many eccentric mannerisms, and almost no capacity to look after herself. After a year's stay, she could wash and dress herself, do her own washing, and go to town for shopping or to collect her pension.

The residents selected to live in long-stay hostels were very different from those in the short-stay hostels. Nearly all the residents (94 per cent) had previously had a diagnosis of schizophrenia, and they had stayed in hospital for a much longer period of time (50 per cent for over 20 years as opposed to only 12 per cent of the short-stay group). They also tended to be more socially isolated: two-thirds had no friends at all, and only one-quarter had visited a friend in the community in the last month. They were a much older group of people (69 per cent over 55) and much less active; nobody was working full time, and only 12 per cent had part-time jobs.

The selection policy for the long-stay hostels was clearcut. The residents were drawn entirely from the old long-stay mental hospital population, who would have spent the rest of their days in hospital had they not been given the opportunity to live in the community. It should be remembered, however, that they were all living many miles away from their previous homes, and that most of them had very little contact with anyone living outside the hostel. It was unlikely that any of the residents would move on to live a more independent life. Most would stay there until they died.

Group homes

Objectives

By the mid-1960s much concern was being expressed over the usefulness of the short-stay hostel. It was clear that they were highly selective and geared to the needs of those with the greatest chance of living independently in the community. Yet hospital staff could see many people whose acute psychotic symptoms had remitted long ago, and who remained in hospital mainly because there was nowhere else for them to go. They were not acceptable in hostels because they needed permanent rather than temporary accommodation and, in any case, they did not meet the criterion of employment potential. On the other hand, although they had usually spent a long time in hospital (they were mostly part of the old long-stay population) they were fully capable, with sufficient preparation, of looking after themselves with the minimum of staff support. What they needed was an environment where a small group of three to five former patients could live together and give each other friendship and support needed to live outside hospital. What was required, in fact, was to create 'artificial families' for a group of people who had lost contact with their own. This is what group homes were created to provide.

The group-home 'movement' developed very rapidly. Local Associations of Mental Health run well over 150. Many psychiatric hospitals have networks of group homes attached. One of the pioneers, Littlemore Hospital, has more than ten. Housing associations have sprung up in many areas in order to provide more. It is impossible now to say how many there are.

Setting up a group home

To establish a successful group home requires the co-ordination of several different 'resource groups'. First, the medical, nursing, social work, and occupational therapy staff of the local hospital need to be aware of the need. Nurses and occupational therapists are most familiar with the day-to-day functioning of patients and are well placed to help psychiatrists with selection and preparation. Social workers, through contact with Social Services and Housing Departments, are best placed to negotiate for the accommodation and supervision resources that will be required once the selected group of patients moves out into the home.

It is important that the various 'resource groups' involved should meet regularly so as to co-ordinate their various contributions. A steering committee is the simplest way to achieve this. For example, the steering committee for one hostel was composed of four people. Two members of the local Rotary Club were responsible for co-ordinating with the Housing Department, and for finding an appropriate house, arranging for a lease, and providing furniture and fittings (including fridge, washing machine, and vacuum cleaner). A new bathroom was added, which was paid for by the local Association of Mental Health. In the initial stages the main function of the Rotary Club was to ensure that the accommodation met an adequate physical standard and that it was adequately furnished. After the home was established their function tended to be the provision of pleasant 'extras', such as subsidizing the Christmas dinner and decorations. The

General Secretary of the local Council of Social Service was responsible for co-ordinating the contributions of the local community groups. For example, he arranged for Task Force to do the initial cleaning of the house. Later on, he became the administrative co-ordinator. If, for example, one of the local community groups had agreed to provide some furniture, but had delayed, he would chase them up. As Chairman of the Steering Committee it was his responsibility to convene and chair the meetings. The last 'key person' in this particular steering committee was the local authority social worker with special responsibility for group work. In the early stages, she had primary responsibility for the selection and preparation of residents while they were still in hospital; later on for the transition from hospital to the community and for co-ordinating the supervision once the group home was established.

In other cases, community nurses or doctors have taken the leading role. A steering committee is not the only way of ensuring co-ordination between the various agencies. One psychiatric hospital took the initiative by establishing a fortnightly Rehabilitation Committee meeting. This was attended by representatives of the local authority Housing and Social Service Departments, as well as members of the hospital Community Nursing Unit and Occupational Therapy Department. The co-ordinating role in this case was played by a psychiatrist with special responsibility for rehabilitation. He had primary responsibility for selecting prospective group home tenants. The Occupational Therapy Department taught them the necessary practical skills (shopping, cooking, cleaning, etc.). The Community Nursing Unit supervised tenants once they had left hospital. An important role was played by the Housing Department. The fact that representatives attended the rehabilitation committee regularly ensured that they had early warning whenever a house was needed. This enabled the Department to select from its housing stock the most appropriate house available in terms of size and location. Prospective tenants who had not previously lived in the borough were not excluded: 'It would be an intolerable burden on the hospital and indeed on the people concerned who wanted accommodation in the area, if we were to apply a strict geographical demarcation . . . the hospital is in our borough and if people are coming from it, then as far as we are concerned they are now the responsibility of our borough, irrespective of their borough of origin prior to being admitted' (Housing Department co-ordinator).

Effective co-ordination machinery is essential to any successful group home scheme. This implies regular contact between all the staff involved in provision of group home care, whether they are in housing or social service departments, hospitals or voluntary bodies, in order to make sure that the resources available are contributed in a co-ordinated and reliable way, at the time when they are needed.

Selection of residents

The selection process in a group-home scheme reflects the assumptions and preferences of the staff involved. Two different methods of selection have been used: self-selection and systematic selection by staff. One hospital which preferred self-selection began by briefing hospital ward staff to talk to individual patients about the plans for the group home. A few weeks later an open meeting was held for any patient interested in the possibility of starting a group home. About 25 patients attended. The first meeting turned out to be one-sided; staff provided a lot of information about living in the community but few questions were asked and most patients seemed uninterested. However, at the next meeting a week later, all the 15 patients who attended seemed much more interested and asked many questions. Where would they live? How would they manage? What would happen if they didn't like it? Would they miss the hospital? The following week seven or eight patients came. Of these, five decided that they would like to live together in a group home. The advantages of the self-selection system is that it capitalizes on the motivation of patients who wish to make a success of their move. However, difficulties arise from the fact that unsuitable patients may volunteer and that, after one or two homes have been established, there may not be many self-motivated patients left. For these reasons, a rather more formal selection procedure is usually adopted.

The experience of one of the group-home 'networks' in the 1976 study is typical. For the first group home, established in 1972, selection was informal. Nursing staff were asked to put forward the names of patients who were thought likely to be able to live in group homes. Seven patients were suggested and all accepted. The same procedure was adopted for the second group home but this group made a poor adjustment outside hospital. Consequently, the selection procedure for the third group home was more systematic. Forty patients were submitted for consideration by the group-home selection committee on the basis of case summaries provided by the psychiatrist. The selection committee consisted of the psychiatrist, the community nurse who was assigned to the group home, the head of the Occupational Therapy Department, and the occupational therapist concerned with preparation for discharge. All 40 patients were interviewed, as well as ward staff who had special knowledge of the patients concerned. Eight patients were finally selected.

One problem that all selection procedures will encounter is that of the suitable but reluctant patient. It is understandable that someone who has lived for a long period of time in hospital will look upon it as home and be reluctant to consider leaving. This leaves staff with a difficult dilemma: to what extent should patients who do not want to leave be 'pushed' into a group home, in the hope that, in the long run, they will be better off? Another problem in selection concerns the question of underactivity. It is well documented that underactivity leads to an increase in the 'clinical poverty syndrome' (poverty of speech, emotional flatness, slowness, poor motivation, and social withdrawal). A supervisor who visits a group home perhaps for one hour a week can have very little influence on the level of activity in the home. There is nothing to prevent a resident from lying in bed every day if that is what he or she wants to do. To what extent, therefore, should patients with a history of underactivity in hospital be excluded from admission to a group home? A group-home preparation unit in hospital (or attached to a hostel) allows a period of observation during which the answers to these problems usually become clear.

When a vacancy occurred in a given home, the remaining residents were often reluctant to have anyone new come in. In several cases, supervisors decided not to admit a newcomer because the balance and cohesion of the remaining group would have been destroyed. In one home the supervisor selected someone who she thought was highly suitable, but the residents refused to allow the applicant to come for a trial weekend. All the supervisors agreed that filling a vacancy was one of the most difficult aspects of their task, and had to be done with considerable patience and delicacy: 'Immediately after a newcomer has moved in I visit two or three times a week to discuss with them all how things are progressing. A particular difficulty is helping the newcomer establish a role in the house. Often the "old guard" are reluctant to let the newcomer do anything at all, and I have to make specific suggestions like "Why doesn't Anne do the shopping today?" '

Preparation of group-home tenants

For most of the 'old long-stay' a successful adaptation to living in group homes is impossible without thorough and careful preparation in the coping skills they will need to exercise once they are living outside hospital. One hospital which was supporting three group homes ran a 'Daily living' programme for prospective tenants. It was organized by the Occupational Therapy Department with a view to enabling patients to prepare themselves for life in the community. Every week-day morning, a group of three or four patients, sometimes accompanied by a member of the occupational therapy staff, would go to one of the local shopping centres. Each group would buy the food it needed in order to prepare the following day's lunch. They planned the menu and the shopping list themselves. Each person took it in turn to go into a shop, buy the appropriate food, and check the change. They would then return by public transport. Those that had difficulty in travelling would be helped, encouraged, and supported by the others. In the afternoon they could choose to attend a wide variety of classes varying from typing, shorthand, English, and arithmetic, to cooking lessons, Yoga, pottery, needlework, dress-making, and beauty care.

Once the initial selection for the next group home had been made, the selected tenants would 'graduate', after successfully completing the Daily living programme, to the group-home preparation unit. Here, together as a group, they would collectively learn to 'keep house' by undertaking the necessary cooking and cleaning. An OT helper was allocated to supervise them in this stage of preparation. Initially, they would attend the preparation unit during the day, and then return to the wards at night. After a while, however, they would also sleep in the unit.

Characteristics of group-home tenants

During the 1976 survey, 39 tenants living in eleven group homes were interviewed. Compared with short-stay hostels, tenants were older (90 per cent over 45), more often women, had spent much longer periods in psychiatric hospitals, and were more likely to have been given a diagnosis of schizophrenia. Two-thirds had been living in the group homes for more than two years and three-quarters wanted to go on living there. There was, however, little difference in the proportions going out to fulltime or part-time work. Very few group-home tenants attended day centres (3 per cent, compared with 23 per cent from hostels), presumably because there was little encouragement (and supervision) from staff to do so.

In other respects, group-home tenants were similar to short-stay hostel residents. They were 'homeless single persons'. They were just as socially withdrawn but less overactive, demanding or odd in behaviour, consistent with their being older and less recently having had a breakdown. The amount of contact with the local community was limited in both groups; fewer than 20 per cent had visited a friend or relative during the previous week, and 23 per cent had had no such contact for at least six months. Eighty-four per cent had gone out by themselves during the previous week but only 38 per cent had done so in the company of a fellow resident.

Supervision of group homes

Most supervisors in the 1976 survey had reservations about the amount of support available to tenants. Two of the three networks visited had regular meetings at which supervisors met tenants but in the third there was nothing of this kind. An unqualified worker could feel very isolated: 'Nobody in the office knows what you're doing so there's no pool of experience to learn from. I tend to feel out on a limb without any idea of how the set-up as a whole is working.' Volunteers also had little supervision.

Supervisors tended to visit regularly but infrequently; during the day rather than in the evenings. In many group homes, all the unemployed tenants would gather together when the supervisor called. It was quite difficult to get them to talk about personal problems. 'They positively dislike talking about anything personal in the present. For example, someone had given Megan a black eye, I couldn't possibly ignore that and tried to get the group to talk about what had happened. They were angry with me for mentioning it. It took them a long time to talk about it.' Another supervisor commented: 'It's hard to differentiate my role from the volunteers. I've asked the group if they want me to continue to come.'

In part, this sort of difficulty arose from the very brief time that supervisors spent in the group homes. In one network of three homes, one supervisor spent an average of three hours per week in each, which allowed very little time for sorting out personal problems. Tenants did not necessarily help each other. One supervisor commented: 'Sometimes they resent having to help each other. If Jim is ill in bed, sometimes they'll all go out and leave him by himself.' Another supervisor said much the same thing: 'If one of them is going through a bad patch—hallucinating or being very withdrawn—they'd rather pass the responsibility on to me. For most of them, taking responsibility for themselves is as much as they can manage; they don't have any energy left over really to help each other.'

All the supervisors emphasized that a key part of their work was to maximize the independence of residents: 'I have to remember that it's their home and, when I go in, I'm there as their guest.' This meant resisting, if possible, attempts on the part of residents to get the supervisor to take their decisions. One supervisor had great difficulty in resisting tenants' pressure for her to choose the new cooker. However, it should also be said that tenants of another group home said that their supervisor was quite put out when they bought an electric fire without consulting her. Supervisors differed among themselves as to how much of a check they kept on the tidiness of the tenants' rooms. Some regarded the rooms as 'sacrosanct', others always looked in each room on every visit and made 'suggestions if anyone's room isn't tidy.'

In case of interpersonal difficulties, 'my role is to provide a feeling of safety, which enables them to sort it out themselves. When something really difficult crops up, *they* engineer a group meeting.' Often however, it was not that easy: 'Peter would hear voices telling him he'd committed some murders. He'd go along and report it at the local police station. The others felt very embarrassed and felt Peter was letting them down. The police didn't mind (they were used to it) but the residents did. It was very difficult to get them to talk about it but eventually they did.'

None of the supervisors thought that there was much social activity among the tenants. 'The atmosphere there is flat. There's not much communication between them. Half of them stay in their own rooms.' 'There are long periods of silence when they just sit around the room, not doing anything. I feel awkward when this happens when I'm there but they don't seem to mind.' However, there were regular cooking, cleaning, and shopping chores to be done every day, and as long as these were successfully completed there was little real cause for concern about the low level of social interaction.

Nursing supervisory staff were careful to check medication while social work supervisors tended to leave this to others.

The environment as seen by group home tenants

Group-home tenants were asked for their impressions of relationships with others, the quality of life in the houses, and the role of staff and their comments were recorded. Twice as many were favourable as unfavourable. Some examples of each kind, taken from all three networks studied, are given below.

POSITIVE COMMENTS

I understand my background a bit more since I've been here, and the way I approach people.

We all get on very well here. I would hate to go back to hospital.

It would be lonely here if we didn't have each other.

I'm always glad to come back here. It's lovely to be home.

We get up when we want to. Joyce and I get up together and have cornflakes and tea for breakfast.

We do the washing between us. The home help comes in to help keep the dining room tidy and that sort of thing.

Everyone gets as much attention as they need.

If you have got any problems then they are prepared to help you, providing you tell them.

He's more like a brother than a social worker. He's one of us. He comes and looks after us. We have a laugh and joke with him.

NEGATIVE COMMENTS

I object strongly when Linda cleans her teeth in the kitchen and won't do the dishes.

I have very little social life here. The rooms are too small. You have got to plan to invite your guests here when the others are out.

One sizes up what she [the social worker] wants to hear. One does not say what she doesn't want to hear.

If you are not feeling well, all the others can say is, 'I'm sorry you're not feeling well' . . . they don't feel things very deeply.

I don't know him [the social worker] very well. I don't talk to him. I haven't got anything to say to him.

There is nothing very much for us to do round here. There are no pubs nearby.

Comparison of hostels and group homes

It is plain that the residents of hostels and group homes differ in important respects, although there is some overlap. Hostels nowadays tend to take younger people, earlier in the course of psychiatric disorder, and without a long history of hospital residence. Group homes are set up for the more chronically handicapped. Nevertheless, both groups share the characteristic of being 'homeless single persons' and it may be that some residents of hostels would be better off in group homes and vice versa. Three criteria are particularly important in judging the effectiveness of the two kinds of environment: autonomy, quality of life, and cost.

Autonomy

Residents in group homes report that just over half of all decisions about which they were asked were taken on their own personal responsibility, compared with just over one-third for hostel residents. Two of the hostels placed a good deal of emphasis on joint decision-taking while, in the other two, most decisions were taken by staff.

Decisions in group homes supervised by social workers tended to be taken more often by tenants than in group homes supervised by community nurses. This may be due to the closer supervision by community nurses, who visited twice or three times a week, compared with social workers. There is also a possibility that the network of homes supervised by nurses contained more handicapped people. The influence of professional attitudes also needs to be considered.

Quality of life

The first mental hospitals were set up, nearly a century and a half ago, in order to provide a better quality of life for mentally ill people than was available under the conditions of community 'care' available at the time. The same claim is now made for residential alternatives to hospitals. Quality can be assessed in terms of participation in community affairs, richness of interpersonal contact, degree of autonomy, and degree of satisfaction.

Neither hostels nor group homes can be said to be 'part of the community', any more than local hospitals, in the sense that residents participate in the same way as most members of ordinary households. Hospitals that are situated outside the areas they serve are, of course, at a disadvantage in this respect, as are hostels similarly placed. 'Participation' depends mainly upon employment, but very few hostel or group-home residents are, in fact, employed.

Social contacts within hostels and group homes are not very close. More than half (53 per cent in the 1976 survey) are limited to brief formal conversations with staff or fellow residents. This may be due to the fact that many residents are socially withdrawn following attacks of schizophrenia. Hospital studies have suggested that underactivity is harmful and can be counteracted but it is common in hostels and in group homes. Nearly half the hostel residents and nearly two-thirds of the group-home tenants had no job and did not attend a day centre. Hostel staff made no intervention in respect of nearly half the problems they described as due to social withdrawal.

Costs

In 1976, costs per resident week varied, in the hostels, from £41.96 to £61.21. The largest single factor was staff salaries (51 per cent to 82 per cent). Although rents paid by residents covered only a small proportion of the costs (12 per cent to 20 per cent) they were nonetheless quite high. This meant that centrally funded supplementary benefit provided a hidden subsidy to local authorities in respect of unemployed residents.

Group-home costs were much lower, Network 2 was nearly self-supporting in terms of running costs (£1.11 per resident week). Staff salary cost per resident week was £1.08.

Family care and boarding out schemes

In an early article on family care, J. K. Wing summarized its advantages as follows:

The system is claimed to be economic, because hospital bed space is released, the cost per patient may be less, and the patient may be able to do valuable productive work; humanitarian, because of increased privacy, freedom, dignity, and responsibility; social, in that the gap between society and the patient is more easily bridged; therapeutic, since there may be good opportunities for treatment, rehabilitation and eventual discharge.

The same author commented: 'Family care has never been a feature of English psychiatry except in the form of guardianship' (3000 mentally retarded patients were being cared for in the community, many in foster families). Family care has proved a much more popular form of provision in Europe.

Boarding out as an alternative to hospital care has until recently received little attention. Gregory reported that the Ministry of Health recorded only 47 patients as boarded out in 1964, and 76 in 1967. Rolf Olsen commented that 'These estimates, although rightly conveying the overall picture, are grossly inaccurate in that a number of institutions were by this time boarding out, and by the end of 1967 the North Wales Hospital had itself placed 174 patients in boarding houses.' Recently, however, boarding-out schemes have become more popular. In 1976, the National Association of Mental Health held a conference on the subject and the ensuing report recorded 27 schemes currently operating. Seven of the schemes had provided a total of over 1200 placements. If it is remembered that the total number of hostel places available in 1975 was only 4500 it is clear that boarding-out schemes are at last beginning to make an important contribution to after-care.

Many different methods have been used to locate landladies; broadcasting on the local radio, writing articles and advertising in the local papers, and going round town on foot knocking on doors. Occasionally, insufficient landladies have been found to make the scheme worthwhile. The more typical experience, however, has been to receive too many offers of help. This has particularly been the case in tourist areas where seasonal fluctuations in business have rendered the possibility of a steady all-the-year round income particularly attractive. Consequently many new schemes are faced with the difficulty of deciding which landladies are suitable and which are not. That this can be a complex process is illustrated by the experience of Rolf Olsen, who found that a number of landladies who volunteered for the boarding-out scheme of the North Wales Hospital had recently been widowed, and they themselves needed supportive counselling. When this was given, they withdrew their offers to help in the scheme. This illustrates Olsen's argument that,

of prime importance [in selecting landladies] was the motivation of the person wishing to be responsible for the patient's care . . . it was important to identify and enable those applicants with motives that did not seem likely to meet the patient's needs to be able to recognise this for themselves and to withdraw from the scheme. If they did not withdraw then to refuse application.

Olsen also found that it was useful to interview the landlady's family. This was because he felt it was important that each member of the family should be informed as to the demands and difficulties that might be involved. He commented: 'Those groups with members who did not inter-relate satisfactorily, did not agree to the undertaking, or who saw the arrangement as a way to resolve their own personal difficulties, were rejected', adding that

it was important to determine the level of expectation held by the applicants about the patient's behaviour, likely performance and capacity to form satis-factory relationships. This was found to vary considerably between those who had a consistently low expectation, with a belief in the need for excessive control and authority over the patient, to those who held a too high expecta-tion and failed to recognise and accept that some patients would show aspects of behaviour, for example, a lack of cleanliness, poor eating habits or irrational behaviour, which they would find unacceptable.

Lastly, the physical standards of the house were carefully examined, and guide-lines laid down. The understanding was that there should be 'at least three meals a day, that no more than four persons should share one bedroom, that each patient had his own storage space, that the house should be centrally heated, hot and cold running water in each bedroom, a minimum of one bathroom to every ten persons, and that there should be a sitting room available to the patients at all times.'

All personnel with experience of running boarding-out schemes agree that supervision of the landlady is as important as supervision of the client. Usually, the person with overall responsibility for running the scheme will supervise all the landladies, whilst delegating respon-sibility for supervising the clients to individual social workers. (In north Wales, however, the social worker was responsible for super-vision both of the client and the landlady.) As with the group homes, the usual practice has been to visit both client and the landlady fairly frequently in the early phase of placement, and then to visit less regularly once the placement has stabilized.

The experience of the north Wales boarding-out scheme illustrates the importance of regular and consistent supervision over an extended period of time: 'At the beginning of the discharge policy regular multi-disciplinary case conferences were held with all appropriate hospital and local authority workers, including psychiatrists, nurses, psychiatric social workers, mental welfare officers and welfare officers, to discuss the scheme and select patients for discharge.' A social worker would then discuss the discharge proposals both with the patient and the relative and would then keep the monthly conference informed of the progress made. The Psychiatric Social Work Department sent a monthly report to the relevant officers in the five counties of North Wales, informing them of patients discharged. However, after the first year of operation, the system of monthly co-ordinating conference began to peter out. This led, in Olsen's view, to seriously detrimental consequences:

the discontinuance of the conferences led to a profound breakdown in inter-departmental communication at field level which was compounded by the significant lack of co-ordinated planning at a policy level . . . The result of the breakdown in communication at both administrative and field levels was that the hospital continued to develop the policy of boarding out patients without the continuing approval and support of the local authorities, and without anyone assuming the responsibility of co-ordination and oversight. Given this situation, antagonism and conflict between the local authorities and the hospital was inevitable and it began to show itself in deteriorating relationship between the staff of the institutions concerned and to make itself known in the adverse press reports which appeared.

In the Manchester Social Services boarding out scheme, landladies are encouraged to charge slightly higher than the going rate for ordinary lodgings. This acts as an incentive and also helps the department build up a sizeable group of landladies. They are encouraged to rent out all their available rooms. Up to £157 can be spent on redecorations or furniture for a room made available by a landlady. These fitments then remain the property of the Social Service Department. In the Croydon Social Service Department, a retaining fee is available which can be paid for up to three months on rooms where the patient is not yet ready to move in or where a former patient has had to be readmitted to hospital for up to three months. The department also underwrites landladies for any damage done to their property by ex-patients in their care.

In the north Wales scheme, all the landladies thought they were underpaid (£5–£5.75 per resident week in 1966) for the work and responsibility involved. This was a contributory factor towards the landladies recruiting the maximum possible number of patients, even to the point of overcrowding.

Olsen suggested that the key issue in assessing the success of boarding out schemes is whether they serve simply to relocate psychiatric patients in community instead of hospital wards, or whether they can serve an additional function in alleviating chronicity. He makes the case for the latter function as follows: 'boarding out schemes provide the opportunity to return to and be supported by the community, personal family-based care, employment, increased privacy, greater self-determination, a greater dignity from the opportunity to contribute to their own and the well-being of others as opposed to the passive acceptance of institutional care.' He concludes, with respect to the north Wales scheme, that 'with important reservations these objectives were successful and that they offered a viable alternative which has many advantages over hospital care. In particular, they enabled the patient to return to the community . . . a greater degree of privacy and independence, and opportunity for self-determining behaviour, as well as the chance of an increased dignity from the possibility to contribute to the well-being of others'.

Discussion

Several important issues arise from this review of studies of non-hospital residential accommodation for the 'adult mentally ill'. None of them can completely be resolved on the information available but tentative judgements can be made and all deserve further investigation.

The first issue concerns the nature of the need for residential accommodation. This is part clinical, part social. Most users of hostels and group homes, particularly those who stay for six months or more, share with long-stay in-patients the characteristics of 'homeless single persons'. This term is usually applied only to people who live in lodging houses or shelters for the destitute but it is useful, in understanding the provisions needed, to see what the groups have in common. They have little contact with relatives, few social supports, no means to pay for accommodation, and are frequently handicapped. There is often a background of social disadvantage and a long history of unfavourable self-attitudes. Such people are more likely to be admitted to a wide variety of residential settings.

The disabilities of the group are also varied though not as severe as those of long-stay hospital patients. Those in MACA hostels and in group homes, on the whole, were representative of the less handicapped among what has been called the 'old long-stay' hospital population. Those in group homes were middle-aged to elderly, predominantly female, socially isolated and unoccupied. Three-quarters had been given a diagnosis of schizophrenia. (The MACA group had these characteristics in even greater intensity, except that the sexes were more equal). Over half had been resident in the home for more than two years and three-quarters wanted to stay. They were withdrawn but not seriously demanding, unstable or bizarre in behaviour. Staff thought that three-quarters had a lasting impairment and would probably need sheltered accommodation permanently.

Preparation units for group homes have been established in hospitals and at least one is attached to a local authority hostel. Once a tenant is established in a group home, however, there is little opportunity for influencing behaviour except by exhortation because supervisors rarely have more than 20 minutes a week, on average, to devote to any one person. This leaves a great deal of autonomy to tenants but also allows a great deal of inactivity. Two-thirds in the 1976 survey had no occupation apart from their contribution to the housekeeping. It may be that this is the best environment for disabled people who are unable to meet everyday stresses but it is important that a follow-up study should be conducted to make sure that deterioration does not occur because of understimulation. It is not clear, for example, why more tenants could not have attended a day centre.

Family care and boarding out are other options for this group. Each could be used more than it is. Much depends on skill in selecting families or landladies and in continuing supervision. Attendance at a day centre, where feasible, allows a good deal of unobtrusive supervision.

Short-stay or 'rehabilitation' hostels take a much more mixed group. Some residents appear to be similar to those in group homes. Some are more handicapped or disturbed, selected from the 'new long-stay' hospital population. Others present rather different problems; they are younger, more often men, more active and demanding, and have diagnoses such as neurosis or 'personality disorder'. It must be quite difficult to create a social atmosphere that is ideal for all these groups at once.

Without more specific evaluative studies it is impossible to comment on the effectiveness of the rehabilitation techniques used in short-stay hostels. It is, however, clear that, even in hostels chosen because of their good reputation, most interventions by staff are not of a highly skilled nature, and that the kinds of 'technical' interventions used vary a good deal between hostels. A *lack* of intervention was particularly evident in respect of behaviours such as social withdrawal, poor performance, overdependence, and underinvolvement, which accounted for nearly half of all those reported as problematic by staff.

Most hostels are not restrictive in the sense used by Apte but the tenants of group homes experience a good deal more autonomy. The comments of hostel residents were about equal in commending a relaxed atmosphere and in suggesting that more structure and pressure should be applied. If the aim is indeed to settle the residents in less supportive accommodation it would appear that a planned 'course' of rehabilitation should be available, those who do not respond being considered, after a year or so, for other types of setting. When half-way houses were first set up there was very little alternative accommodation available. Now the option of moving to a group home or to a supervised bed-sitter or lodgings might be more routinely considered. The possibility of setting up some group homes where there is a higher degree of supervision also requires consideration and experiment.

A consideration of costs reinforces this conclusion. Clearly, if exposure to a high-cost rehabilitative regime does result in the resident becoming independent, there should be an overall saving compared with group homes. However, many residents in hostels have stayed for more than a year and would like to stay for longer. This does not make economic sense.

A further possibility that deserves serious consideration is that rehabilitation (particularly vocational training but possibly 'resocialization' as well) might more often be carried out in day centres, one or two of which already exist in most local authority or hospital areas, rather than in hostels.

This raises a further problem; that of the co-ordination of residential and day care services, whether provided by hospital, local authority, or voluntary organizations. The underlying principle is that all mentally disabled individuals living in a defined geographical area should be regularly assessed in order to consider whether their current setting is the one most appropriate for them. This would include all those living for more than six months in psychiatric hospitals, hostels, group homes, bedsitters, and lodgings (and also disabled people living with their own families), thus automatically including day attenders as well.

There are formidable organizational and management problems since the agencies involved include hospitals, social service departments, housing authorities, employment officers, and a range of voluntary bodies. The assessment procedures adopted by each agency should include common elements. Above all, there should be a common review procedure, perhaps co-ordinated by an officer of the social services department. The primary task of any joint committee set up to make decisions would be to match the people needing accommodation (wherever they happened to be living at the time) to the facilities available, and to put forward bids for new services as necessary.

Such an arrangement would help overcome the isolation of many existing units and foster the creation of one responsible, comprehensive and integrated mental health service.

FURTHER READING

Apte, R. Z. (1968). *Halfway houses*. Occasional Papers on Social Administration, No. 27. Bell, London.

Clark, D. H. and Cooper, L. W. (1960) Psychiatric halfway hostel: a Cambridge experiment. *Lancet*, **i**, 588.

DHSS (1975). *Better services for the mentally ill*. Cmnd 6233. HMSO, London.

Hewett, S. H. (1979). Somewhere to live, In: *Alternative patterns of residential care for the discharged psychiatric patient*. (Ed. R. Olsen.) BASW, Birmingham.

— Ryan, P. and Wing, J. K. (1975). Living without the mental hospitals. *J. soc. Policy*. **4**, 391–404.

Mann, S. and Cree, W. (1976). 'New' long-stay patients: a national sample of 15 mental hospitals in England and Wales, 1972–3. *Psychol. Med.* **6**, 603–16.

Olsen, R. (1976). Boarding out the long-stay psychiatric patient. In *Differential approaches in social work with the mentally disordered*. (Ed. R. Olsen.) BASW, Birmingham.

Ryan, P. and Hewett, S. H. (1976). A pilot study of hostels for the mentally ill. *Social work today*. **6**, 774–8.

— and Wing, J. K. (1979). Patterns of residential care: a study of hostels and group homes used by four local authorities to support mentally ill people in the community. In *Alternative patterns of residential care for the discharged psychiatric patient*. (Ed. R. Olsen.) BASW, Birmingham.

— and Brown, G. W. (1970). *Institutionalism and schizophrenia*. Cambridge University Press, London.

5 Providing for the destitute

John Leach

The historical background

An historical examination of social responses to destitution[1] indicates that poverty has long been regarded as due to deliberate laziness, to be deterred by punishment except in a few deserving cases. The inflexible policies adopted by central and local government as a result of this assumption were completely inappropriate to the disparate needs of those labelled as paupers or vagrants. During the reign of the Tudors vagrancy was widespread and the government, in an attempt to eradicate it, introduced severely punitive policies. Between 1569 and 1572 the Privy Council undertook a 'whipping campaign' against vagrants. Repeated vagrancy was a capital offence. This repressive legislation had little effect on the number of vagrants and the government attempted to reduce the problem by providing work for the poor. This aim remained central to government thinking and during the eighteenth century workhouses, in which paupers could be concentrated, were built to facilitate it. Thus began the policy which was to reach its culmination in the Victorian era.

By the early nineteenth century the expense and inefficiency of poor relief had resulted in widespread demands for reform. In 1832 a Royal Commission was set up to enquire into the problem and its deliberations resulted in the Poor Law Amendment Act of 1834 (the New Poor Law). In order to deter 'incorrigible' vagrants, it was enacted that the condition of those receiving relief was to be made less eligible than that of the lowest paid labourer, and that relief should be given only in workhouses. Conditions in these workhouses were frequently appalling.

The last two decades of the nineteenth century witnessed the beginnings of Poor Law reform. In part, this reflected the impact of investigators such as Booth and Rowntree (who showed that poverty was not necessarily synonomous with indolence), in part the growing influence given to the working classes by the extension of the franchise. In

---

[1]Destitution is defined here as prolonged inability to pay for accommodation other than that available in reception centres and shelters.

1905, as a result of the changing climate of opinion, a Royal Commission on the Poor Law was set up. The Minority Report of the Commission, anticipating the Welfare State, suggested that the Poor Law should be replaced by specialized social services dealing with separate categories of poor people.

It was not until 1930, however, that the administration of poor relief was taken over by local authorities. This coincided with a period of economic crisis, and high unemployment swelled the ranks of the destitute. Vagrants filled casual wards and cheap lodging houses all through the 1930s. With the outbreak of the Second World War and the abatement of mass unemployment, the numbers in casual wards fell to a few thousand.

After the war, under the National Assistance Act of 1948, authority for dealing with the destitute was vested in central government. Government policy was to provide 'reception centres' where 'persons without a settled way of life' could be provided with temporary accommodation while needs were assessed and long-term placements arranged. Since accommodation would be temporary, it was believed that the evils of the old mixed workhouse would be avoided. Those administering the centres thought that destitution would rapidly be eradicated. They assumed that the post-war welfare legislation would eliminate poverty and that pockets of hardship would only persist because of personal disability or special need, which could be dealt with by the other services of the Welfare State. This optimism led the National Assistance Board, in 1948, to close 156 of its 290 casual wards, and to plan for further reductions in its accommodation.

In the years that followed 1948, however, there was no evidence that destitution was declining to any large extent. The problem, in fact, attracted growing attention and the mid-1950s witnessed the first of a large number of post-war surveys of destitute groups. It is necessary to consider the findings of these surveys before discussing the question of provision.

The characteristics of the destitute

Post-war surveys of the destitute have been primarily concerned with persons frequenting reception centres, common lodging-houses, and free shelters. These groups are to some extent interchangeable. The destitute often move from one form of accommodation to another and, on occasion, sleep rough. The great majority are men. The most authoritative estimate of frequency was provided by the National Assistance Board's *Homeless Single Persons* survey in 1966, in which

567 establishments for the single homeless were included. These establishments provided 31 932 beds, 27 512 of which were occupied on the night of the count. On the night of 6 December 1965, 2800 sites known to be used by men who slept rough were visited, and 920 men counted. These numbers were probably an underestimate but nevertheless provided evidence that the problem of destitution had not gone away.

A survey of the largest reception centre by Tidmarsh and Wood in 1971 provided information about the characteristics of its users. These men tended to be born into large families in areas of social and economic deprivation, such as Eire, Scotland, and the North of England. Their fathers were often unskilled manual labourers and their childhood was spent in poor, overcrowded living conditions. They left school as early as they could and acquired no vocational skills. Being unable to find work many moved to areas where employment might be easier to obtain. They moved from job to job, pursuing single-sex occupations such as labouring work and kitchen portering. Most never married, either because they found it impossible to maintain any kind of settled home in the midst of continual poverty and occasional unemployment or from disinclination. In these circumstances, they were unable to save money, tended not to contribute to pension schemes, and were quickly out of pocket when they became unemployed. A high proportion had been charged with offences connected with alcoholism and vagrancy. Even when working at their best these men were in a financially precarious situation, and any crisis, such as an accident or illness, could precipitate destitution. The onset of destitution usually occurred in middle age, but more recently, the age of onset has been getting lower, possibly reflecting the depressed state of the economy and increasing unemployment.

The health of these men is often poor. An Edinburgh survey of men living in common lodging-houses who attended a general practice showed that they were referred to hospital after consultation three times as often as other patients. Chronic bronchitis, pulmonary tuberculosis, and malignant disease were common. In a survey of tuberculosis mortality in England and Wales in 1968, six common lodging-house residents were found to have died of unrecognized tuberculosis or to have been admitted to hospital in a moribund state.

Mental disabilities are also common among these men. The Edinburgh general practice survey found gross psychiatric illness present in 12 per cent of the men, and chronic alcoholism in 9 per cent. In another survey Priest, a psychiatrist, found that a definite psychiatric condition was present among Edinburgh common lodging-house residents as follows: organic brain disease 7 per cent, schizophrenia 26 per cent, depression 5 per cent, alcoholism 9 per cent, personality disorder 12 per cent, and subnormality 8 per cent. Fourteen per cent of this sample had previously been in mental hospitals. Priest made the point that these diagnoses were of the more severe psychiatric disorders with the prevalence of schizophrenia being particularly high.

Surveys of the men living in government reception centres have revealed a similar morbidity. A survey of the Camberwell Reception Centre, the largest statutory agency, found that the hospital admission rate of schizophrenia from the Centre was eight times that of the male population of London. A one-night census of the Centre in 1965 showed that a quarter of the inmates had been admitted to a mental hospital. A further quarter were alcoholic. The survey by Tidmarsh and Wood categorized the interviewed men's conditions into one of ten categories according to the investigator's judgement of the predominant problem suffered by each man. From this it was estimated that nearly a quarter of the 'new cases' attending the centre during the course of 1970 had, as their predominant problem, a mental illness. Twenty-nine percent of the men interviewed in this survey had been in a mental hospital; 9 per cent within the year prior to interview. Surveys of reception centres in other parts of Britain show that Camberwell's high psychiatric morbidity is not unique.

Findings of this kind have led research workers to suggest that both statutory and non-statutory provision failed to meet the needs of the destitute. This view was shared by a number of emergent voluntary organizations, which, during the 1960s, saw their role as establishing a completely new kind of service. The assumptions made by these organizations, and the outcome of their attempts at rehabilitation and resettlement, shed light on the problems that have to be overcome if adequate provision is to be made.

The voluntary response

The Simon Community, the most influential of the new organizations, was founded in 1963. 'Simon' staff, while recognizing the importance of material relief, believed that the destitute also possessed pressing non-material needs. These were seen as emotional or psychological in nature. They could be met, the Simon volunteers believed, through a policy of fostering close emotional bonds and egalitarian relationships between helpers and helped. The word 'community' was adopted by the organization to emphasize the fundamental importance of these considerations.

This philosophy was based on a belief that social isolation and a fear of relationships, arising from inadequate personality development, was the basic problem of the destitute. Destitution was seen as a reflection of 'inadequacy' and the destitute were regarded as the victims of a competitive, impersonal society. They could best be helped, the volunteers believed, in a setting that replaced prevailing social values.

The alternative values put forward were strongly influenced by Christian ideals. The voluntary workers rejected materialism and expressed a 'willingness to see Christ in even the most abandoned character'. Some writers, in support of these ideas, equated destitution with other-worldliness and saw the life-style of the destitute as a manifestation of fundamental Christian values. The role of the communities, according to people who believed this, was twofold. It was to befriend and shelter individuals whom they regarded as vulnerable and persecuted and to join, with them, in creating a distinctive way of life.

Brandon has described the initial approach of one such Community. It was established in 1971 to house destitute women. 'Some of us were interested in applying ideas of "beingness" culled from Buddhism and Gestalt therapy to a residential setting. What would happen if you didn't treat people as problems to be solved? If you rejected the labelling that had taken place in the wider community?' The Simon Community, with similar general aims, attempted to create a therapeutic environment completely accessible to its clients. To this end the Community took over, in 1967, a former rag storage warehouse located in an East End street inhabited by crude-spirit drinkers. These men were encouraged to sleep in the warehouse and were allowed to bring their drink on to the premises.

The staff of these Communities explicitly rejected the procedures employed by the statutory agencies. Within reception centres inmates are required to undergo an interview and a process of cleansing and disinfestation. Such procedures, the voluntary workers suggested, were humiliating and unproductive. They alienated the destitute and made them reluctant to ask for help. Within small communal hostels, on the other hand, a permissive, informal environment was seen as a prerequisite for 'rehabilitation'. The hostel's role was one of 'social treatment', in that its regime was the therapeutic agent. Hostel staff believed that the experience of destitution encouraged an adaptation to particular values and modes of behaviour. Since it might be too stressful to discard these immediately, an environment should be provided which would mediate between the previous life-style of the destitute and the demands of the community.

In assuming that social treatment would effectively facilitate resettlement, the advocates of this approach did not consider the effect of disability. It has been noted that there is a high prevalence of physical and psychiatric illness among destitute men. The problems that this was to cause hostel staff can be illustrated by the experience of three London half-way hostels studied by Hewett and Ryan. The hostel residents had been discharged from psychiatric hospital. The majority were without family support and earned low incomes. They would have had, after leaving the hostels, to compete for accommodation in a situation of severe housing shortage. The researchers pointed out that the standard of living the residents could afford to buy on the open market would have been much lower than the one they had become accustomed to in the hostel. The goal set for this group was one of moving into isolated bed-sitting rooms. Once there they would need to meet unaccustomed responsibilities such as paying bills, preparing food, maintaining their medication, and getting themselves up for work. Even allowing a considerable measure of rehabilitation, such a goal would be very difficult to achieve.

Hostel residents who have been destitute will confront similar problems. Many will be severely handicapped and most will be socially isolated. They will face a recurrence of destitution upon discharge if they are unable to cope with the problems of independent living because of residual handicaps and a lack of resources. The staff of hostels are, in any case, often reluctant to admit people of 'no fixed abode' on the grounds that they will have nowhere to refer them if rehabilitation is successful. In consequence, appropriate hospital referrals are rarely made for this group. The policy of early hospital discharge advocated by the 1959 Mental Health Act has resulted in these patients alternating between hospital residence, reception centres, lodging-houses, and sleeping rough.

Page, who worked at the Camberwell Reception Centre, cited a typical client: 'I think of one schizophrenic, aged 39, whose life during the past four years (since he left hospital after an eight-year stay) has become a shuttle service between reception centre, prison, and hospital. He lives in a dream world of his own. His latest "crime" was the appropriation of a teddy bear.' Another man had spent 15 years in a mental hosptial suffering from schizophrenia before taking up residence in a Salvation Army hostel. 'He had been in the hostel for six months when interviewed and was dirty and unshaven. He was incapable of caring for himself and had no knowledge of necessary current affairs, such as Social Security benefits. His sole possession was a child's spinning top. He is sent to the Cleansing Station to be disinfested regularly as he is incapable of washing himself or his clothes and the hostel does not consider it to be part of its function to rehabilitate people.'

It is against a background of gaps in community provision for the handicapped that the policy and operations of voluntary and statutory resettlement services should be viewed. Page saw the ressettlement policy of reception centres as unworkable since it presupposed a non-existent level of community provision. The extent of this deficiency is apparent from a consideration of the provision available for one destitute group, those suffering from alcoholism.

The extent of alcoholism among the destitute has already been indicated. In 1971, the problem of habitual drunken offenders (many of whom are destitute) was considered by a Home Office working party. Under Section 91 of the Criminal Justice Act, 1967, the abolition of imprisonment as a penalty for being drunk and disorderly is provided for. It is stipulated, however, that this charge should not be made until the Home Secretary is satisfied that sufficient suitable accommodation is available in the community for the care and treatment of the persons convicted of the offence. The working party attempted an assessment of the services that would be needed if Section 91 was to be implemented.

They concluded that the facilities required would need to be adequate to cater initially for 2000 male offenders and that subsequent users, over a period of a few years, might more than double this figure. Having predicted demand, they estimated the number of suitable community services then in operation. At the end of 1969 only 10 hostels for alcoholic offenders, providing between them 92 places, had been approved as suitable for a Home Office grant. Hospital provision for alcoholics did not compensate for this deficiency. In 1971 there were 13 alcoholism treatment units attached to psychiatric hospitals. One, in the North of England, had taken in only two destitute men for treatment, during the year ending July 1971.

The shortage of facilities for homeless alcoholics has resulted in much of the work in this field being pursued by voluntary organizations. The Alcoholics Recovery Project, for example, used 'shop fronts' (small, informal meeting-places situated in skid-row areas of London) which vagrant alcoholics were encouraged to visit in order to discuss their problems with no strings attached. ARP also provided small hostels in which alcoholics, contacted through the shop fronts, were offered residence.

Central government and local authorities have established links with the voluntary organisations that bear the brunt of this work. In 1973, for example, Lambeth Social Services Department offered ARP the role of agent in developing alcoholism services in the Borough. To this end they provided the organization with a grant, in order to fund the salary of an extra social worker. Similarly, contacts between ARP and Lesisham Council have resulted in a working party on the problem and the hope of some practical action.

Attempts at resettlement

Statutory and voluntary organizations have experienced common difficulties in resettling the destitute, arising from the effects of disability. This has occurred despite differences in ideology and approach. The experience of a statutory and a voluntary organization will be considered briefly in order to illustrate this situation.

The statutory agency is the Camberwell Reception Centre. This is a large institution, built in the 1870s, and mention has already been made of the disabilities suffered by many of its clients. The survey by Tidmarsh and Wood showed that those with alcoholism or a mental or physical illness stayed for longer periods than those without illness or handicap. Eighty-eight per cent of those without a medical impairment attended for less than one week, compared to 43 per cent of those with a mental illness. The mean number of nights spent at the centre in one year by different groups of men were as follows: no medical impairment—5 nights; alcoholism—27 nights; physical illness—46 nights; mental illness—48 nights. The centre, while operating within a framework which emphasized the provision of temporary accommodation, was faced with a situation characterized by chronic handicaps. Its function, a depository for the disadvantaged irrespective of their particular needs, was that of the nineteenth-century workhouse.

This dilemma is not unique to the statutory services. It has affected voluntary organizations, among them the St. Mungo Community, a charity which derived much of its approach from the Simon Community. St. Mungo's provided a soup run, which it used to contact men sleeping rough in London, and a number of small houses which served as permissive, communal hostels. Destitute men, contacted on the soup run, were taken into residence in the houses but usually left again very rapidly, resuming their life on the streets. Men only began to settle in houses after a process of assessment was adopted, in which men staying in a St. Mungo night shelter were systematically considered for admission to a house. The group who settled in the houses had experienced prolonged destitution and as many as a half were also severely handicapped. Psychiatric disabilities were particularly prominent.

The St. Mungo experience, therefore, was similar to that of the

Camberwell Reception Centre. Both organizations, because of the accumulation of handicapped men, were unable to maintain a flow of men from the streets back to independent life in the community. Paradoxically, success in contacting the destitute meant stagnation. About one-third of the men in the St. Mungo houses could have moved to less supervised accommodation, such as bed-sitters or group homes, if these had been available. Only by providing additional services of this kind could a movement of men through the organization be maintained.

Providing for the destitute

In considering provision for destitute men it is useful to distinguish two overlapping groups. In the first group, destitution occurs largely because of social disadvantages such as a scarcity of accommodation and employment. This explanation is insufficient, because most people from such backgrounds do not become destitute, but there is often no other obvious factor, except a postulated (and not very helpful) condition of 'inadequacy'. In the second group, however, obvious handicaps have contributed to destitution. Terms like 'rehabilitation' should presumably carry different implications in the two groups, but the distinction is rarely made. Thus one school of thought (often supported by the staff of voluntary organizations) suggests that most destitute people are 'inadequate' because the structure of society has left them no other option. The social treatment of a caring community is therefore aimed at correcting adverse social experiences, thus enabling the men gradually to regain their self-respect and, subsequently, their social competence.

This theory is influenced by the belief that poverty and destitution are two sides of the same coin. If this is the case, preventing one would also prevent the other. However, as we have seen, the ultimate experience of voluntary organizations has been similar to that of reception centres; a large proportion of their clients have severe handicaps as well as a long history of social disadvantage.

Studies that have concentrated on people accumulating in accommodation specifically designated for the handicapped have *begun* with these problems. They have demonstrated that, among these groups, there are often chronic impairments which, although they can be made worse by adverse social influences, still persist even when the social environment is as favourable as it can be made. In this sense, they are 'intrinsic'. The chronic impairments that sometimes accompany schizophrenia are an example (see Chapter 2). The social disadvantages that many of these people had suffered, long before they ever showed symptoms of schizophrenia or other diseases, can be termed 'extrinsic'. The terminology is not important but the distinction is.

The model of rehabilitation on which this discussion is based, is developed in Chapter 9. It is sufficient, for our purpose, to consider the implications of the distinction between intrinsic impairments and extrinsic disadvantages for a policy of resettlement. People who are both destitute and suffer from severe impairments will require supportive day or residential environments. Since the degree and nature of impairment will differ from individual to individual, and since some people will progress or relapse, the kind of support required will be very variable. An effective network of services would therefore have to comprise diverse yet co-ordinated facilities, with easy movement within or between them.

The fact of scarce resources emphasizes the need to clarify the areas in which facilities should be concentrated. This discussion will conclude by considering three complementary kinds of service urgently required by the destitute. The first kind facilitates contact, the second is residential, the third provides specialist help.

Contact with the destitute is a necessary preliminary to resettlement. It is often difficult to achieve due to the unsettled nature of this population and its heterogeneity. Particular kinds of service will attract some destitute groups but not others. A variety of facilities is therefore desirable.

Most of the work in this field has been undertaken by voluntary bodies which have attempted to provide basic help (material and psychological) without undue conditions or formality. Night shelters, soup runs, and day centres have been organized with this end in view. Observation of the work of these services suggests some comments which might be of use to the volunteers manning them. For the sake of simplicity the discussion will be restricted to the work of night shelters. Most of the guidelines, however, apply to contact services in general.

Contact services providing shelter for the destitute must aim to attract as many men as possible. To achieve this, informality and permissiveness is essential. Men should be able to use the shelter free of charge and without having to undergo a formal procedure (such as an interview), although staff will find it useful to enter names into a register in order to provide a record of those who use the shelter regularly and might therefore be willing to move to a more permanent form of settlement. Restrictions on drinking and strict adherence to times of opening and closing should be kept to a minimum. Too much red tape, if enforced, will result in the exclusion of men who would otherwise have used the shelter.

A policy of this kind will obviously present some problems. Some men get drunk, become difficult to control and exhibit aggressive behaviour. Staff often have to ask them to leave for that night. Such men, however, comprise a small minority. Most want peace and quiet and a chance to get some sleep. They appreciate a regime that provides a degree of security and order. Instances of aggressive behaviour usually diminish after an initial period of contact, during which the staff's willingness to enforce rules is tested. This occurs because destitute men often view those providing them with services as two-faced. 'They're all sweetness and light until we get out of line', was the way one man expressed it. If this attitude is to be changed, rules should be administered with fairness and consistency, and the reasons for them explained. A man should not be penalized on the basis of his past record. These responses are crucial in establishing a good relationship. If a man considers a social worker, nurse, or volunteer helper to be 'straight' (whatever his view of the rules they enforce) a basis for trust is provided. This is the first step in any plan of help.

Many of the men staying in the shelter will not, however, express a wish for help, nor show any desire to interact with staff. Some will prefer the company of other shelter residents, others will remain solitary and talk to no one. Attempts at contact with either group, with the aim of assessing needs and attitudes, can be protracted and frustrating. It might involve no more than a few minutes strained conversation every few days, concerning the weather, places suitable for sleeping rough, or the varying quality of the shelter soup. The man may mumble his replies, avert his gaze, and speak only if a question is put to him. Interaction can continue on this level for months, and in some cases will never progress. It should, however, be continued, as far as possible, since it forms the basis of any future attempt at help. It is important, therefore, that there should be a group of full-time staff who use their time to build up relationships with the men and are responsible for supervising the work of less experienced volunteers. They need the patience and perception not to force the pace of the relationships that they make. Many men will have been destitute and socially isolated for years. Changes in their attitudes are unlikely to occur quickly.

Because of the wide variety of physical and mental disabilities exhibited by destitute men, shelter volunteers are greatly helped in their work if they have access to medical and social-work personnel who can advise on the management of problem cases. If possible, some form of regular liaison should be established. A doctor based at a local hospital, a GP, or a nurse, might be prepared to spend a few hours a month operating a surgery at the shelter. Such work is of service to the men and can be of general benefit in increasing communications between the shelter and the area's health services. A social worker prepared to work in an informal consultative capacity could perform a similar role. Senior shelter staff should make every effort to initiate such contacts.

These services allow the assessment of need and provide information and advice. Some clients, of course, might not want to be rehabilitated. A night shelter or soup run might be the only kind of settlement they are prepared to accept. Irrespective of this, the relief that such services provide clearly has a humanitarian value. In time, also, some habitués might become amenable to the idea of a more settled environment.

Contact facilities tend, by nature, to be makeshift and unsophisticated. The Simon Community's adaptation of a warehouse into a shelter for crude-spirit drinkers is an example. The potential to expand this provision, without a prohibitive increase in resources, is therefore considerable. The inner cities, where the destitute tend to congregate, contain many premises which would be suitable as contact centres. The St. Mungo Community, for example, adapted a large derelict factory, situated in Vauxhall, for use as a night shelter. Within a few months it was accommodating 100–200 men nightly, many of whom became regular users. The same organization, with virtually no resources, began a nightly soup run staffed by a few volunteers. Initially the soup was made from vegetables begged from a local market.

Contact services function in a vacuum, however, in the absence of accommodation to which those who use them can be referred. The scarcity of accommodation in the community has already been noted. At present, there is no likelihood of the services for the destitute achieving a suitable placement for the majority of their clients.

Two kinds of residential provision are required if this situation is to be remedied. The first would consist of cheap lodgings, of an acceptable standard, for single working men earning low incomes. The closure of many common lodging-houses, and a decline in the rented housing market (traditionally the sector used by the low-wage earner), has precipitated an impoverished but otherwise settled group into destitution. Increasing unemployment has exacerbated this situation by inflating demand for a declining supply of cheap accommodation.

An increase in cheap lodgings would not, however, meet the needs of those who are handicapped as well as homeless. This group requires supportive accommodation. Within such accommodation (usually a small hostel) staff attempt to provide a home for their residents. The concept of a home refers to an informal environment in which each member participates and to which each feels he belongs, because of strong bonds of friendship and mutual concern. Many men requiring residential care, however, are quite unable to contribute towards this social interaction, or even to contribute much to day-to-day household chores. This throws a large part of the initiative on the staff.

Staff should make every effort to foster relationships with the residents. Daily life in a small environment offers many opportunities for this. Men should be encouraged to speak about their feelings and express their likes and dislikes (for example, about meals, television programmes, the colour the living-room wall is to be painted, and so on), since this increases a sense of belonging and participation. Similarly, the expression of individual interests should be stimulated. One man, in a hostel for destitute men in west London, spent most of his time doing nothing until it was discovered, by chance, that at one time he had enjoyed gardening. He was encouraged by the staff to dig over a small piece of disused land at the back of his house and plant flowers and vegetables. He found the activity immensely rewarding.

Staff should try to speak to each resident every day, especially if some men are withdrawn and solitary. This ought to be possible in a small hostel. Regular conversations (even if, on occasion, they only involve a few minutes chat after breakfast or supper) help to persuade the residents that staff have a continuing interest in their welfare. This encourages frank discussion of problems and helps prevent the occurrence of sudden crises. Often, such crises are sudden only in the sense that staff have lost touch with the feelings of the individuals concerned.

An important role of staff is to mediate between residents during disputes. These are inevitable in small, communal environments and, if not controlled, can result in quarrelling, bullying, and general unpleasantness. Daily contacts with all residents should provide staff with advance warning of disputes and potentially serious situations can often be defused by speaking privately to the parties involved. If staff find it necessary to arbitrate they should make every effort to be consistent and fair, despite their personal preferences for the individuals concerned. Other residents should have the right to discuss and question the decision.

Staff are sometimes surprised at the contribution of handicapped and uncommunicative men to the running of the hostel. Sometimes, lack of resident participation is less a matter of skill than of confidence. The task of staff is to increase and sustain confidence and, to this end, every resident should be encouraged to engage in some level of hostel management. Tasks need to be chosen which will challenge the resident without being beyond his present capacity. Some residents, if staff encouragement and support is sufficiently strong, will find their own role. A resident of a St. Mungo hostel who was brain-damaged and unable to express himself coherently, made the kitchen his preserve, did much of the washing-up, and kept the cooker and sink-unit clean. He took great pride in this work as he did in running errands for a fellow resident who had a heart condition and was sometimes incapacitated by severe fits of depression.

Residential provision for these men, as for others with handicaps of comparable severity, ought to be provided by the health and social services. Social service departments, however, are reluctant to provide supervised accommodation for the severely handicapped. Most of the hostels provided for the mentally ill, for example, are occupied by people without severe handicaps. This difficulty is compounded when patients of 'no fixed abode' leave psychiatric hospitals even though accommodation there is judged appropriate for them, It has been suggested that hospitals should set up supervised hostels using health service funds and this is being done in a few centres. This will make little impact, however, on the problems facing agencies which work with the destitute, since many of the handicapped men accumulating in their accommodation have not wanted to stay in hospital and have no wish to return there. It was pointed out in Chapter 1 that much of the current philosophy of psychiatric hospitals is against using them for long-term care and opinion seems unlikely to change in the near future. Given this situation, there is no alternative to trying to provide the destitute who are handicapped with a decent form of supervised accommodation in the community. This accommodation will need close links with the health and social services. Developments currently taking place in this field indicate the kinds of initiative that are required.

Contact services such as shelters and soup runs need some kind of medical back-up to their work. A Manchester night shelter, for example, was visited regularly by a mobile surgery, manned voluntarily by two local GPs. Over 300 people were treated during a six-month period. Following this experiment arrangements were made to register shelter residents as temporary patients at a local health centre. Occasional visits to the shelter were made by doctors treating those too sick to attend the regular surgery. At the present time efforts are being made to establish a surgery at the shelter itself.

A similar initiative was made by the St. George's Mens' Care Unit of the Methodist East End Mission in Tower Hamlets. The Mission established a nursing service, the male nurse involved giving his time voluntarily. For those needing the care of a doctor, a back-up GP was involved in the project.

At the level of supportive residential accommodation, more permanent links should be established with the health services, both at general-practitioner level and at that of the community psychiatric nurse based at the local psychiatric hosptial. The work of the St. Mungo Community shows the value of such an arrangement. This organization established links between two of its hostels and their local psychiatric hospital. A community psychiatric nurse visited the hostels regularly, saw some of the residents and discussed them with the hostel staff. Many of the residents were receiving psychotropic drugs and some had regular injections of fluphenazine, in order to prevent a relapse of schizophrenia. Readmission to hospital, when necessary, was facilitated by this liaison, and the staff were very pleased with it.

Innovations of this kind form the pattern for the kind of service that ought to be available to the destitute, as to others with similar disabilities. The deficiences of the welfare services, however, affect those with few social roots or resources far more than those with family or friends. Extra services are necessary to compensate for these deficiences. At present, the services provided for the destitute are inadequate. There is, however, considerable potential for change. Given the resources, the effectiveness of action depends on two conditions. The first involves an acceptance of what resettlement means and entails. Until this is appreciated an effective network of services cannot be established. The second involves the agreement of priorities. Some areas in which resources can usefully be concentrated have been indicated. There is need for a greater number and variety of contact services. Their work should be supported by residential facilities in the community, including unsupervised lodgings, group homes, and hostels. Both contact and residential facilities should have an adequate liaison with wider health and social services. The effectiveness and co-ordination of these services should be routinely evaluated and their role reassessed.

The very number of innovative, shoe-string services that have been established to help the destitute, allows, if only in one sense, a measure of optimism. Much can be done with very little. The dedication of many workers is our only abundant resource. If this idealism could be harnessed to an overall plan of action, based on a clarification of priorities, much could be acheived. There is an urgent need for such an approach, and for the resources to sustain it. The problem of the destitute has not gone away, nor is it going.

FURTHER READING

Archard, P. (1975). *The bottle won't leave you*. Alcoholics Recovery Project, 47 Addington Square, London SE5.
Brandon, D. (1974). *Homelessness*. Sheldon Press, London.
Cook, T. (1975). *Vagrant alcoholics*. Routledge and Kegan Paul, London.
Edwards, G. et al. (1968). Census of a reception centre. *Br. J. Psychiat.* **114**, 1031–39.
Hewett, S., Ryan, P. and Wing, J. K. (1975) Living without mental hosptials. *J. Soc. Pol.* **4**, 391–404.
Leach, J. and Wing, J. K. (1979) *Helping destitute men*. Tavistock Publications, London. To be published.
National Assistance Board (1966). *Homeless single persons*. HMSO, London.
Page, P. (1965). Camberwell Reception Centre. *New Society* **134**, 18–21.
Priest, R. G. (1970). Homeless men—a London survey. *Proc. R. Soc. Med. 441—5*.
Steward, J. (1975). *Of no fixed abode*. Manchester University Press.
Tidmarsh, D. and Wood, S. M. (1972). Psychiatric aspects of destitution. In *Evaluating a community psychiatric service. The Camberwell register 1964–71*. (Ed. J. K. Wing and Anthea M. Hailey.) Oxford University Press. London.
Wood, S. M. (1976). Camberwell Reception Centre: a consideration of the need for health and social services of homeless single men. *J. Soc. Pol.* **5**, 388–99.

Information on benefits

The disability rights handbook for 1978 can be obtained from: Disability Alliance, 5 Netherhall Gardens, London NW3 5RJ. Price 60p or 75p by post.

6 Caring for the mentally retarded

Lorna Wing and Judith Gould

This chapter is concerned with the group of mentally retarded people who are likely to need supervision and protection all their lives. They include almost all children and adults who are severely retarded (intelligence quotient below 50) and a minority of the mildly retarded (intelligence quotient 50–69). It is written for professional workers and relatives who are involved in caring for mentally retarded people, whether in their own homes, in hostels, or in hospitals. We have concentrated upon practical rather than theoretical problems. The limitations of space have made it necessary to deal with many issues briefly and superficially, but the list of further reading at the end of the chapter provides an introduction to what is now a very useful literature.

In the United Kingdom, the prevalence of the types of handicaps mentioned above varies from about 3 up to about 5 in every 1000 children aged under 16, and around 2 or 3 in every 1000 adults. These figures are based on the numbers of mentally handicapped people who are cared for by the services for severe mental retardation. The overall prevalence rates and the rates for the different patterns of handicaps to be described in this chapter vary from one part of the country to another, although the size of and reasons for these variations are, as yet, unclear.

The problems faced by families with handicapped relatives result from a combination of many different factors. These include the parents' social class, education, material circumstances, their intelligence and personalities, and how many other major difficulties they have to cope with in addition to the handicapped child or adult. The most important factor of all is the nature of the handicap itself. A non-mobile child with cerebral palsy, for example, has many needs which are quite different from those of a hyperactive, destructive, non-communicating child, or from a young adult with good social skills, but no ability to read, write, or count, who is becoming aware of how much less competent he is than others in his age group.

Mental retardation is a general term that covers many patterns of handicaps, each of which can occur in varying degrees of severity. The type of handicap is closely linked to overt behaviour and to the kind of education and management that is required. Although it is an over-simplification of a complex situation, it is possible to classify retarded people into two major divisions, that is mobile and non-mobile, each of which can be subdivided into four groups, depending on the patterns of handicaps. We shall first consider methods of helping and counselling in relation to these eight sub-groups, and then discuss the special needs that all mentally retarded people and their families have in common. A schematic outline of the eight sub-groups is shown in Table 6.1.

Table 6.1 Sub-groups based on patterns of handicaps in the severely mentally retarded

Mobile	Non-mobile
(a) Evenly retarded in all skills	The same sub-groups as for those who are mobile can be observed but the physical handicaps tend to dominate the picture.
(b) Visuo-spatial skills especially severely impaired.	
(c) Language and social communication absent or especially severely impaired.	
(d) Communication present, but social interaction markedly abnormal.	

Patterns of handicaps

Mentally retarded people who are mobile

Mobility can be defined as the ability to walk without any help, and to be able to manage stairs with no, or the minimum of, assistance. The four groups of handicap patterns seen among mobile retarded people are: first general retardation affecting all skills more or less evenly without marked behaviour problems; second, severe impairment of visuo-spatial skills; third, absence or severe impairment of language and social communication; and, fourth, marked abnormalities of social interaction. The groups overlap with each other with no sharp cut-off points, but it is helpful to consider each separately in order to under-stand the needs of those who have the problems in typical form and those on the borderlines.

It is possible to work out to which of these groups an individual child or adult belongs by asking people who know him well to describe his skills, deficits and behaviour, by considering the results of psycho-logical testing, and from direct observation. The descriptions we shall give of each of the groups will be a guide to classification.

(a) General retardation affecting all skills more or less evenly. This pattern is the most common one, and is seen in the majority of the adults who live at home with their own families. People with Down's syndrome (the proper name for mongolism) are especially likely to show this picture of even retardation, except for their tendency to be clumsy in all motor skills, including speech.

Children and adults in this group are, on the whole, easy to get along with, once it is understood that they are backward. Their behaviour is fairly predictable, because it resembles (though is not identical with) that of a normal person of equivalent mental age.[1] The 10-year-old evenly retarded child with intelligence quotient of 40 and a mental age of approximately 4 years is less creative, more restricted in behavioural repertoire, and much slower in learning than a 4-year-old normal child, but the differences are of degree rather than kind.

Children like this tend to follow the same paths in development as do normal children, but at a much slower pace. Those with intelligence levels in the severely retarded range usually cease developing when they reach a mental age of approximately 5 or 6 years, though some go a little further and some do not reach this level. They may have poor articulation and other kinds of speech problems, but, like normal children, they have imaginative pretend play, when they reach the relevant mental age (round 20 months); that is, they begin to hold dolls as if they were real babies, to brush their hair, and to pretend to feed them, or they imitate the noises of cars and trains and drive them along imaginary roads and into pretend garages to fill up with petrol. Later on, children play pretend games with each other, acting out mothers and fathers, doctors and nurses, or spacemen and robots. Their social interactions are also appropriate for their level of development.

Since this type of retardation is often associated with Down's syndrome and also with other chromosomal abnormalities, the diagnosis may be made soon after birth, or at least within the first year of life. If the parents accept the child and decide to bring him up within the family, they will have to come to terms with the slowness of his physical and mental growth. All the difficult phases found in babies and toddlers—weaning onto solid foods, toilet training, and teaching other self-care skills—are drawn out to seemingly interminable length. Dur-

---

[1] Mental age can be calculated by measuring how a child performs on standardized tests of intelligence, and then finding the age at which the child of average intelligence would be expected to obtain the same results. For example, a retarded child of 10 years might score more or less the same as the *average* 5 year old, in which case he could be said to have a mental age of 5 years. These calculations are, of course, only approximations, helpful in giving a rough idea of the level of skill to be expected.

ing the prolonged baby and toddler stages, the parents need much emotional support and encouragement. It is helpful for them to learn from parents of similar older children that progress does occur. A considerable amount of experience and good judgement is needed on the part of the adviser, since some mentally retarded children do remain at a very low mental age and continue to need all physical care. It is difficult indeed to find a way between undue pessimism on the one hand and false optimism on the other.

Retarded children in this group make best progress in a warm and loving family environment in which they can have a wide range of interesting experiences of a kind they can appreciate and enjoy. Parents should be encouraged to take the child on outings, to point things out to him, to tell him simple stories about the things he has done and to find him suitable toys. These do not have to be expensive and complicated. All kinds of household equipment, not to mention empty packets, bottles, and containers of all shapes and sizes can be adapted to give the child practice in fitting things together, building towers, manipulating to improve finger dexterity, and later on, as props in pretend play. The rule here, as in all else, is to consider the child's *mental* age, and to adapt toys, occupations, communications, and general expectations to that level, and not to his physical age.

There is currently much interest in methods of stimulating development in mentally retarded children. Some people believe that special teaching can speed up the learning of self-care and practical skills and, even more important, allow the child to learn more than he would without such help. Some programmes, such as the Portage project (see reading list), give precise instructions geared to the individual child, and require only a small amount of time each day to be given by one adult. Others, such as the Doman–Delacato method of working with cerebral palsy, demand intensive involvement for long periods of time from all members of the family and even outsiders as well. Many people, including the present authors, feel that very heavy demands of this kind are likely to be disruptive for the family as a whole, and it is, in most cases, unreasonable to subject parents to the emotional and physical burden of carrying through such a programme. There is, as yet, no clear evidence that special techniques can help a retarded child to reach higher levels than he would do with ordinary teaching methods though it seems quite possible that they may speed up the acquisition of skills that would have been learnt in time anyway. Even this is worth while, especially in such things as toilet training, self-feeding, washing, and dressing, if it can be achieved by the expenditure of a realistic amount of time and energy, if the parents and the child enjoy the sessions, and as long as the other children in the family also receive their fair share of special attention.

Many teaching programmes use the general principles of 'behaviour modification'. These are, very briefly, the carefully timed and consistent use of rewards for desirable behaviour in performance of skills; the discouragement of undesirable behaviour; and the teaching of skills by breaking them down into tiny steps, teaching one step at a time, and using suitable prompts to help the child perform, which are slowly faded as he improves. These principles are based on a large number of experiments designed to find out the way in which people learn. This brief account leaves out all the useful details. One is the method of 'backward-chaining' whereby the last step of a skill is taught first, and then the penultimate step, and so on, until, finally, the child can carry out the whole process. For example, the last step in putting on a jersey is pulling it down to the waist. Before that comes putting an arm in the second sleeve, before that, putting an arm in the first sleeve, before that putting one's head through the jersey's neck. The first task of all, which is taught last, is arranging the jersey so that, when it is worn, the front is in front and the back at the back. Some books on behaviour modification, written for parents, have now been published, and family counsellors should keep up with these, so that the best ones can be recommended to parents who are interested.

The whole idea of behaviour management has aroused much opposition in some people. To some extent, this has been because some workers have carried the method to extremes, apparently working with children for hours at a stretch, pressing them to perform on tasks beyond their capacity and using punishments such as electric shock. This approach is hard to justify, especially as there is little convincing evidence that it produces better results than a less intensive programme. However, the basic principles of behaviour modification are largely common sense (applied systematically), and have always been known and used by parents as one of the ways to control behaviour and to help the child learn skills. It is possible to use this approach at times when it is appropriate, without having to accept it as the one and only way to solve all problems, and without losing sight of the child as a human being.

As children develop language and the ability to think about things for themselves, so learning and control of behaviour come to depend more and more on discussion and understanding of ideas and a desire to please, rather than simple behaviour modification applied from outside. For this reason, behavioural methods are more often necessary for retarded children than for normal children. Among all kinds of retarded children, those who are evenly backward are perhaps least likely to need such methods to be applied very systematically for long periods of time, but they are useful in the early years and also for dealing with the various behaviour problems that may arise.

These problems are like those of young normal children, but made worse because they last longer and therefore are still occurring when the child is becoming too large to pick up and remove from a difficult situation. They include temper tantrums, destructiveness, stubborn refusal to co-operate, pestering for attention, all of which are likely to be worse in front of visitors or in public. These do tend to fade as the child grows older, but can be diminished in the young child by a consistent, firm approach. The biggest temptation for parents is to give the child much attention when he is being difficult and even to try to placate him with sweets or cuddling. This just makes matters worse. It is best to ignore him if possible, or to remove him from the situation and put him where he can be safely ignored, but give attention and praise when he is behaving in acceptable ways.

An evenly but severely retarded child, when he becomes adult, is usually friendly, sociable, and willing to be helpful to the best of his ability, though he retains the immaturity that is the inevitable consequence of his low mental age. Whether he continues to live with his family or goes into some form of residential care, he will need to be in a protective environment that does not make demands that he cannot meet. While life remains reasonably well-organized and predictable, a severely retarded adult in this group is likely to remain well-adjusted within his limits, but a severe, though uncommon stress, such as bereavement, or some common and fairly minor upset at home, may produce a regression to more childish, difficult behaviour, at least for a time. Parents or other relatives can help by planning very carefully in advance any changes over which they have some control and explaining to the retarded person in a way that he can understand. Of course, this is not always possible. If a behaviour breakdown does occur, the family will need extra support. Such an event may lead to admission to residential care, either temporarily or permanently, as the only solution.

Severely retarded people with an even profile of skills are not usually physically aggressive (though they may learn some choice verbal abuse from their peers at school or training centre). But, because of their immaturity, they may lash out in a fit of temper, especially if they find it hard to express themselves in other ways. This should be dealt with calmly and firmly and, if possible, by removing them from the provoking situation and guarding against recurrence. If aggression, or window-smashing, or other violent behaviour occurs fairly frequently, ways of preventing or coping need to be discussed and agreed with the parents, the training-centre staff and anyone else involved. The advice of a psychologist skilled in behaviour management should be sought if possible. This type of problem seems to reach a peak in adolescence and early adult life, but to diminish with age. Sadly, it may not be possible to prevent and it is one of the major reasons for a request for hospital care.

Delinquent or criminal behaviour is rare in severely mentally retarded people. The supervision they require makes it difficult for such behaviour to occur. There may be petty stealing from parents or from other people at the school or training centre, because the immature person finds it hard to resist obvious temptation. The best way to deal with this is to put food and money away out of sight, locked up if necessary, and to supervise as closely as possible to make sure that such petty crimes are always detected and the spoils returned to their owners. Calm firmness without too much fuss is again the most helpful approach.

One of the major worries of parents of retarded adolescents and adults is how to cope with the young person's sexual feelings and interests. Physical sexual development occurs quite normally in most retarded people, and those who are socially aware, as are the group being discussed, are likely to feel attraction towards other people of the opposite, or, sometimes, of the same sex. It can happen that a physically attractive but severely retarded girl is exploited by an unscrupulous man, or that an adolescent retarded boy finds himself in trouble because he makes immature and inappropriate advances to a girl, or else is led into homosexual encounters because of his naivety.

There is no simple answer to these problems. Parents should be encouraged to explain the facts about sex as far as their child can understand and will need to repeat the explanation many times. Parents also need to be reassured that masturbation is natural, normal, and has no harmful consequences, though they will need to teach their child that it is done only in private. Use of the contraceptive pill or other suitable contraceptive methods as a safeguard in girls who, because of their behaviour, are at risk of becoming pregnant is a sensible precaution, as long as the parents and the girl herself are happy about the idea. There are now medications available to reduce the sex drive in men though in many cases the main problem is the social behaviour rather than excessive sexual drive.

There has been much more open discussion of the sexual needs of handicapped people in recent years. Some workers in the field feel that mentally handicapped people should be allowed to marry if they want to do so, and that the mental subnormality services should provide suitable accommodation for couples. In some places, this has been tried. Sometimes the unions are stable and successful, in other cases not.

While this arrangement can be a most happy solution for some people, it is not, in practice, possible for the great majority of severely retarded adults. There is no real answer to the problems caused by sexual drives in these people, except understanding, supervision and acceptance of any substitute sexual activities that are not harmful or distressing to others. In this area, more than any other, the beliefs and emotions of parents or caring staff are very much involved in their reactions to the handicapped person's behaviour, so it is hard to lay down any rules.

Retarded people can have episodes of psychiatric disorder, such as anxiety, depression, mania, or schizophrenia, which may last for only a short period, although in some they become chronic and long lasting. These episodes may occur in response to some life event, and sometimes can follow a feverish illness such as influenza. It may be that retarded people are more susceptible in this respect than people of normal intelligence. It is always worth considering the possibility of a superadded psychiatric illness when a retarded person shows a major change in behaviour. Because the symptoms are likely to be childish and bizarre in form, the true nature may be overlooked or explained away as being due solely to mental retardation. If such illnesses do occur, the advice of a psychiatrist experienced in this field should be sought.

(b) Severe impairment of visuo-spatial skills. This group of retarded people develop social skills and understanding of language to a markedly higher level than their ability to co-ordinate movements and to deal with spatial problems such as fitting shapes together or remembering the shapes of letters and numbers. When these latter skills are severely impaired, the person concerned has difficulty in learning to dress, because he cannot figure out how to put his clothes on the right way round, he is clumsy in many practical tasks needing good co-ordination, and he is likely to have difficulty in all kinds of school work, including reading, writing and craft-work. He may have difficulty in articulating words because this is a skill requiring muscular co-ordination.

Children like this are socially responsive especially within the family, they understand language up to their mental-age level and they have pretend-play. In many ways they are like the evenly retarded group and most of the comments and suggestions already made are applicable. However, as they grow older their social responsiveness and interest in other people make them painfully aware of their special handicaps. They want to play games, they want to do jigsaws, to learn to read and write at least as well as their classmates can, and to take part in the art and craft activities, but they are held back by their innate clumsiness.

How they cope depends, at least partly, on their own personalities. Occasionally such a child cheerfully accepts his lot and is popular because of his friendly disposition. More often, children like this become rather shy and do not want to mix with large groups of children, because they are afraid of being knocked down in rough games (a fear based on reality). Some develop marked anxiety and even depression. A number of these children are especially interested in simple patterns made by flickering lights, and even twist and turn their hands or objects near their eyes to obtain such simple sensory stimulation. For this reason, plus the shyness when in a large group, these children may, mistakenly, be called autistic. Their sociability in small groups and their imaginative play show that this diagnosis is quite wrong.

Parents are likely to have problems because of the slowness with which such children learn simple self-care, especially dressing. They never learn to do this without much assistance. They can be helped to put clothes on the right way round by laying garments out on a flat surface, in the correct order, so that, if picked up and put on, the front will be in front and the back to the back. It is, however, a long hard task, and many parents succumb to the temptation and dress the child themselves, because it is so much quicker.

Even with the most skilful teaching, there is no guarantee that these children will make much progress in visuo-spatial skills. It is important for parents and teachers to praise and encourage the child in areas in which he can perform and to be as patient and understanding as possible with his inevitable failures. Some protection from the hazards of boisterous groups in the playground is also necessary, though this should be as unobtrusive as possible.

The impairments last into adult life. The pressures of school no longer apply but, instead, competence tends to be measured in skill in domestic and practical tasks. Unfortunately the person who is poor in visuo-spatial skills tends to fail here also. Much attention has to be given to ways of finding some area in which the person concerned can perform so that he does not feel he is a failure in everything.

(c) Severe impairment of language and social communication. Chil-

dren and adults with this pattern of handicaps are much harder to understand and have many more problems than the two groups described above.

The severe impairment of language affects understanding as well of use of speech, gesture, and all other methods of communication. Most important of all, the child with this type of problem lacks the ability to develop concepts (ideas) of sufficient complexity to allow him to link present experiences with past events, and thereby to anticipate the future. Many do have an excellent rote memory for things they have heard or seen, but this is rather like an exposed film in a camera—that is, an accurate record without any understanding of the meaning.[2] Sometimes people with very poor or no language or social communication have no skills at all, apart from the ability to walk and run and they may be incontinent and need all care. Others, however, are quite good at practical work, self-care, and fitting and assembly tasks such as jigsaws. They may love music and remember tunes very well. These non-verbal abilities may give the misleading impression that they really are quite intelligent and are just refusing to talk. The truth is that their severe impairments make it impossible for them to achieve independence, however good their non-verbal skills. They need more supervision and care than retarded people who are less skilful in non-verbal tasks, but are evenly backward in every area.

The poor ability to think and understand and communicate leads to many behaviour problems. Social interaction is limited to enjoyment of physical contact, or, in some cases, is virtually absent. The children, and the adults as well, who are affected in this way fail to understand even the simplest of the rules that govern social behaviour. There is usually distress at, and resistance to, change. Repetitive routines, or stereotyped movements, such as arm flapping, hand or object flicking, rocking, head banging, or other self-injury are common. Restless wandering, destructiveness, temper tantrums, noisiness, or even screaming are also frequent problems. The children do not play pretend games, and they are very difficult to occupy, since they seem to be interested only in their repetitive activities.

People of this kind may be diagnosed as having an early childhood 'psychosis' and some are classically autistic. These conditions should not be confused with the psychoses usually beginning in adult life, such

---

[2] Some retarded people in the first two sub-groups described above have ideas and imagination appropriate for their mental age level, but have defects of speech. They usually try to compensate by using gesture and miming, and are quite different in behaviour from the sub-group with severe impairment of language and social communication.

as schizophrenia, mania, or psychotic depression. The early childhood 'psychoses' are due to a severe impairment of language and social development. It is to be hoped that some better name will be found for these latter conditions so that they are no longer confused with the adult illnesses. Although it is sometimes argued that such people are not 'really' mentally retarded, in practice they need a great deal of care and close supervision, and the great majority are eventually placed in some kind of mental handicap service.

Education and management of this group presents special difficulties, but some practical suggestions can be made. The first rule is always to make allowances for the difficulty in understanding complex language. It is much easier to convey what is wanted by concrete demonstration. The young children in this group learn motor skills if their limbs are physically guided through the necessary movements. Visual demonstration, simple gestures, and, for the brighter children, drawings and pictures may be useful.

Change is always distressing, so a regular routine and a consistent approach are the ideal to be aimed for (but rarely attained in real life). When new events can be predicted, it is very helpful if some simple way can be found of telling the handicapped person in advance, and making the change as slowly as possible. For example, moving from nursery to school, or school to adult-training centre is made easier if the child is taken on several visits to the new centre together with someone he knows well, gradually extending the time, before he attends permanently.

It is necessary to try to diminish the frequency of difficult, disruptive behaviours and to encourage the development of useful skills and constructive occupations. The carefully planned, firm and consistent approach used in behaviour modification is particularly applicable. The parents can be put in touch with a psychologist experienced in these techniques if one is available in the area. In some areas there are groups led by professional workers that parents can join, in which they can discuss their problems, learn behavioural techniques, and give each other emotional and practical support. Unfortunately, in many places, these services are not available, but books on the subject written for parents are now being published. A family adviser could read and discuss possible methods of management together with the parents.

Children with this type of impairment very often look alert, physically normal, and attractive. If they have some special non-verbal skills, parents (and often professional workers too) tend to believe that the child is potentially of normal intelligence. A few can perform, in some areas, up to the normal level or even above, but most are retarded, many severely or profoundly so. When this becomes obvious, after medical and psychological assessment and observation of the child's development, then the parents should be told about the prognosis and given opportunities to discuss all the implications for the future, many times over if necessary. In particular, a decision has to be made as to whether to seek placement in a special school for autistic children. On the whole, this is helpful for many of the less handicapped children, but those who are also severely retarded are usually best placed in educationally subnormal (ESN) (severe) schools, although the staff need knowledge and experience in order to manage and teach them successfully. The staff–child ratio has to be sufficiently high to allow for some individual teaching and for appropriate management of behaviour problems.

Puberty usually occurs at the normal age. Because of the impairment of social communication, sexual interests are mostly on an infantile or childish level. Masturbation in public is the commonest problem, and needs to be dealt with calmly and sensibly, using behaviour-modification methods if appropriate. The aim is to confine this normal activity to places where it is acceptable, not to stop it altogether. The less severely impaired children sometimes have a childish curiosity about other people's bodies and may try to undress other children, or touch and fondle adults, even complete strangers, in the street. This needs the same calm approach; firmness combined with the minimum of fuss. Unfortunately, inappropriate advances to strangers cause fear and distress in people who are not familiar with mental retardation, and is the type of behaviour quoted when public opposition to new locally based services builds up. It is therefore necessary, as far as possible, to prevent such incidents occurring by careful planning, and supervision and training.

Improvement in behaviour may occur with increasing age, but there can be a difficult phase in adolescence and early adult life. The social naivety and poor communication tend to be life-long. Whereas it is possible to cope with a child like this when he is physically small, the problems of management can become very great indeed when the child grows up and the parents themselves grow older. The family adviser can discuss the possibility of residential care with the parents and arrange for them to visit the places available (see the section on long-term residential care, p. 128). Their fears that harm may come to their child, if he goes away from home, and their feelings that they must not let him down will have to be talked over with tact and sympathy. In the end, only the parents themselves can make this type of decision.

(d) Marked abnormalities of social behaviour. There is a small group of retarded people who appear, on psychological testing, to be more or less equally backward in all areas, but whose social interactions are abnormal and difficult. Some have intelligence quotients in the mildly retarded range, but are placed in schools or adult training centres for the severely retarded because of their behaviour.

They are not aloof to other people as are the group described previously. Many do approach other people, but do so in inappropriate ways. They talk quite a lot but repeat the same few themes over and over again. Repetive questioning, regardless of how many times a full answer is given is quite common. Such people are very tiring to be with, because nothing one can say appears to satisfy them. They talk *at* others and not with them. Other people's interests and feelings are irrelevant to them.

In some retarded people abnormal social behaviour takes the form of explosive outbursts of resentment, rage, and even physical aggression. The cause may be trivial or, on occasions, impossible to determine. These aggressive outbursts may occur in some children and adults who also have repetitive speech. Both of these problems seem to be linked to an inability to understand other people's viewpoints. To some extent this is true of all those with a low mental age, but it is very marked indeed and much more severe than the mental age would lead one to expect in the group described here.

Such children often have a history of placements in several different schools. Their ability to talk quite fluently makes it appear that they have good potential, but their actual achievements in school tend to be disappointing.

There are many problems of management. The repetitive speech can be diminished in quantity if everyone who deals with the child is careful to respond to a remark or reply to a question once only. Repetitions should be ignored, but if the child changes the theme and talks about something new, then he should be encouraged by replying to him. One aspect of this problem which often upsets other people is the tendency in some children for repetitive talking on bizarre or morbid themes, such as murders, monsters from outer space, and so on. A calm refusal to become involved, and as little display of distress as possible is the most helpful way of dealing with these uncontrolled fantasies.

The same repetitiveness tends to appear in the children's play activities. They may go on playing the same simple pretend game over and over again, long after other children have tired of it. Attempts need to be made to introduce new ideas to help the child to join in play with other children instead of following his own preoccupations all the time.

Outbursts of aggression are much harder to deal with. Careful observation may enable the precipitating causes to be discovered. Behaviour modification techniques discouraging the aggression and encouraging more acceptable activities may help, especially if all the professional workers and the parents can carry out the same consistent policy. This is much easier said than done. If aggressive episodes continue into adolescence and adult life, then it may not be possible for the person concerned to continue to live at home, and residential care, most probably in a mental handicap hospital, will be necessary.

Mentally retarded people who are not mobile

All the four behavioural groups described above can be found in non-mobile severely retarded people. As might be expected, profound retardation in every area is more common among the non-mobile than the mobile groups.

The extra degree of helplessness and dependence imposed by the inability to walk by oneself, and all the other problems of feeding, washing, dressing, and toileting tend to take first place when considering the needs of the non-mobile children and adults. Cerebral palsy is also frequently found, and the difficulties imposed by muscle spasm, poor chewing and swallowing, and athetoid movements, add an extra burden.

There is a whole field of expertise that has been developed for managing the details of physical care: designing wheel chairs, hoists, and other equipment; avoiding secondary physical handicaps (such as contractures, bed sores, chronic infections); and encouraging the development of any skills for which there is potential. Advice is available from doctors, nurses, and physiotherapists, from voluntary bodies such as the Spastics Society and the National Society for Mentally Handicapped Children, and from books on these subjects written for parents and professional workers. It is not possible to deal with this very large field in the present chapter. If a family adviser does not have specialized knowledge on this aspect of care, he can still be of help by encouraging the family to seek advice from those with the relevant theoretical and practical knowledge and experience.

Methods of education and management are similar to those for mobile retarded people. The main difference is that parents and teachers have to make more effort and use more ingenuity in devising ways of stimulating and occupying a wheelchair-bound child. Many non-mobile retarded children are so profoundly handicapped in all areas that they are unresponsive to any stimulation, and little can be done except to give them physical care to keep them comfortable. This is by no means true of all the non-mobile group. Some, even though they are severely retarded, are alert and socially responsive and eager for experiences. There are various aids for teaching and for assisting communication if the child has any voluntary movements at all, and it is a rewarding experience to see how much the child appreciates the efforts made on his behalf. Good judgement based on long experience is needed to decide, after a reasonable period of education, which non-mobile child has no potential for improvement, and which one will benefit from specialized help. It is sad that the demands of life make such choices necessary.

Problems affecting all mentally retarded people

Although a variety of different patterns of handicaps can be found among mentally retarded people, many problems are likely to be experienced by them all. These will be outlined here, so that the family adviser is aware of the issues, although it is not possible to go into details.

Reactions of relatives

When mental retardation is associated with obvious physical abnormalities, as in Down's syndrome, the diagnosis can be made soon after birth, or at least within the first year of life. When it is made very early, the first reaction of the parents is one of intense distress and despair and some may not want to keep the child in the family. With sympathetic and realistic discussion, these feelings of total rejection usually pass, except for a very small minority of parents who refuse to have anything to do with the handicapped baby. Where this extreme reaction occurs, even with the most tactful advice and help, nothing can be done except to find alternative care for the child.

In many cases, mental retardation is not confirmed until after the first year. If no problem is suspected for many months or even years, the parents have already become deeply attached to the child, and they have to be helped to adjust their expectations of his future progress.

At the opposite end of the scale from total rejection, and equally undesirable, there are some mothers who become totally involved in the handicapped child, keeping him in babyish dependence and excluding everyone else from the very close relationship. They often develop idiosyncratic ideas of causation and treatment. This can be damaging to the siblings and to the marriage. Sympathetic but frank discussion by an experienced adviser may help, but it is a difficult situation which may never be resolved.

Fortunately, most people are somewhere between these two extremes. There is, nevertheless, always the temptation to over-indulge the handicapped child, partly to 'make up' to him for his handicap, and partly because it is quicker and easier to do things for a child who is slow than to encourage him to do things for himself. A retarded child, perhaps the youngest in the family, can become quite intolerably demanding both at home and in public, unless some sensible rules are laid down and adhered to, just as for a normal child of the same mental age.

It is probably true to say that the brothers and sisters of a handicapped child always experience some disadvantage. This is least severe if the handicapped child is friendly and well behaved. The problems are most obvious if the retarded child is markedly abnormal in behaviour, aggressive, and destroys his siblings' toys and possessions. Such a child may demand so much of his parents' attention that they have no time for the rest of the family.

The adviser can help by being aware of the dangers, discussing them with the parents, and helping them to see that the whole family, including themselves, have needs which must be weighed against those of the handicapped child. Occasional short-term care for the handicapped child can be of great value in achieving a reasonable balance. Sensible advice on managing behaviour and encouraging the development of self-care and practical skills is invaluable in assisting the parents to divide up their time and attention to the benefit of all. Programmes demanding total involvement in the handicapped child alone would seem to be a recipe for disaster if there are other children to be considered, or if the parents want some life of their own.

Discussion groups for parents can be an excellent source of good ideas, and emotional support. A family adviser can discover if any such exist in the local area, or even consider starting one for the families he or she visits.

The voluntary societies set up by parents for various kinds of handicaps have been very successful, both in encouraging the development of services for handicapped people and in the support and interest they give the parents. Some parents find great personal satisfaction in working within a voluntary society even though they obtain no direct benefit for their own child. All families should be told of their existence, and whom they should contact in order to join.

One of the hardest tasks facing professionals who work with the families of retarded children is that of discussing with the family the child's future progress. Every child is an individual, and different from all the rest. Predictions have to be based on what has already happened to other, roughly similar children, not on what will happen to the child in question. Only people with long and wide experience in the field can make a reasonable estimate of the prognosis. The family adviser, even if he is not in a position to do this himself, can discuss the details with the doctor, and then help the family to come to terms with the facts.

Most people need a long time to adjust to the knowledge that their child will never be normal. In a very real sense they are bereaved, and mourn for the normal child they wanted and never had, before coming to accept the handicapped child as he is. Guilt, anger, shame, depression, and anxiety about the future are all experienced in this phase, and may recur from time to time, although the acute pain lessens as the years pass.

Although there are a few parents who never accept that their child is retarded, the great majority, in the end, want to know the truth, even if it is a long time before it is fully faced. Most people are happy if the child does better than predicted, but feel resentful if he does worse than they have been led to expect. The adviser's skill is tested to the full in the task of giving realistic information about the child's future, while still encouraging the parents to believe, quite correctly, that there is a lot they themselves can do to help the child.

Reactions of the general public

Any kind of abnormality in physical appearance or behaviour produces ambivalent responses in other people, consisting of distate and rejection mixed with sympathy and protectiveness. Individuals vary as to which of these two extremes are predominant. On the whole, the former is the more immediate response on first seeing an abnormal child or adult who is a stranger. The latter grows stronger with more personal involvement. Both feelings, however, are equally 'natural' in that they occur spontaneously in everyone. Parents of a child who is clearly abnormal from birth usually go through the transition from the former to the latter, unless they totally reject the child at once.

A family adviser may become involved with trying to change the attitudes of the local community towards handicapped people, either because a family is having problems with a hostile neighbour, or because it is necessary to persuade local residents to accept a new hostel or home for mentally retarded children or adults. In this situation it is worth remembering that the aim is to arouse inherent sympathy, understanding, and desire to protect those human beings who are weaker and less fortunate, and to diminish the automatic hostility to people who are strange and different.

Medication for behaviour problems

Sensible child-rearing, the methods of behaviour modification, and the changes brought about by increasing age, work together to diminish many behaviour problems. Even so, there is a proportion of retarded people, especially those with an uneven profile of development, whose behaviour remains difficult throughout childhood and early adult life.

Sedatives or tranquillizing drugs are often prescribed for disturbed behaviour. These may reduce the level of activity and thereby make the person concerned easier to manage. This result tends to be accompanied by a general slowing up, loss of interest, and often, a marked increase in weight. Sometimes, especially at first, the child or adult is very sleepy and wants to go to bed in the daytime. A diminution in difficult behaviour sometimes occurs when a new drug is tried, or when the dose is raised, but the effect becomes less marked after a time, and a new or additional drug has to be prescribed.

No medication is without its short- and possibly long-term adverse effects on physical and mental state. Parents and teachers are, quite rightly, usually very reluctant to agree to drugs being given. Sometimes it is necessary to accept the lethargy and general slowing up because otherwise the person (usually an adolescent or young adult) cannot otherwise be managed at home or at school.

One area in which medication can be most useful is in coping with the child who keeps everyone else awake at night. This is not particularly common, but, when it occurs, it can have marked effects on the health of the whole family. Night sedation can work very well, as long as the most suitable drug is given in appropriate doses. The prescribing doctor needs to have experience in this field, because some retarded people are very resistant to the level of dosage usually used in people without such handicaps.

Medication is also often necessary for people with epilepsy. Proper control of fits and EEG abnormalities may have additional beneficial results in improving behaviour.

When they reach puberty, many severely retarded girls can be taught to cope with menstruation with a little help, if they are already reliable in toilet training. Physically handicapped or profoundly retarded girls, or those with poor language and social communication, may not manage so successfully and there can be considerable problems if there is no understanding of the need to wear a pad. Where these difficulties arise, hormone pills can be prescribed to prevent menstruation occurring: it is usually suggested that the pills are given for a few months, then withdrawn to allow one menstrual period to occur, then started again, This regime is followed to minimize the chance of undesirable long-term side-effects. It proves very convenient in practice since the periods that do occur can be timed more or less precisely. The same pills are helpful for treating dysmenorrhoea (painful menstruation) or alleviating disturbed behaviour that seems to be related to pre-menstrual tension. In these cases there may be no need to suppress the periods, and the pills are taken for three weeks out of four.

If the girl concerned or her parents are unhappy about the idea of suppressing menstruation for a long time, the hormone pills can be taken to prevent a period just for a special occasion, such as a holiday away from home, if its occurrence would present some problems.

The pills can be obtained only on prescription from a doctor.

Education, occupation, and recreation

The most important aspect of managing behaviour and developing independence in retarded people is the provision of suitable education for children, occupation for adults, and recreation for all ages.

In some areas, there are day nurseries, nursery schools, or nursery classes in special schools which accept pre-school handicapped children. A family adviser can keep up to date with these services and encourage families to use them.

Nowadays, all handicapped children are entitled to education. For some with unusual patterns of handicaps, the problem may be finding the right school. Parents can visit schools and try to find out for themselves which would be most appropriate. Again, a family adviser can help by having full knowledge of what is available.

Day training centres for adults are provided in most areas, at least for people who are mobile and not too difficult in behaviour. Special care units for those who are non-mobile, or profoundly retarded, or difficult in behaviour are beginning to be set up, but are not provided everywhere in the country. Their provision should receive high priority.

Finding suitable recreation can be difficult. Various voluntary bodies, such as the National Society for Mentally Handicapped Children, run clubs for children and adults, arrange outings and parties, and other activities. Information can be obtained from the secretaries of the local society in any area. Horse-riding and swimming are enjoyed by even the most severely mentally and physically handicapped people.

Toy libraries where parents can go to borrow toys for their child, and also to meet each other are being set up in some areas. It is often difficult to know what toys will please a retarded child, and borrowing before buying can save much disappointment and expense. The libraries work best when they are run by people who are experienced enough to guide parents in their selection of toys to try, and to give advice on how to encourage the child to play constructively.

Medical and dental services

Retarded children and adults need general medical and dental care and access to specialized services. They often have associated physical handicaps and epileptic fits. In the United Kingdom, there is no separate, comprehensive service for the mentally handicapped, as there is, for example, in Denmark, so those who are retarded usually have to make use of the same facilities that are available to the general public.

In theory, everyone has the same right to use the National Health Service, but, in practice, this does not always work smoothly. It may be distressing for parents to take a severely handicapped child to the child health clinic where most of the children are thriving, healthy, and normal. Many retarded children are upset by having to wait for long periods and become disturbed in behaviour, to the embarrassment of the parents and the annoyance of other people. The specialist concerned is unlikely to have much experience with mental retardation and may not know how to overcome the difficulties of making a diagnosis and carrying out treatment with someone who is uncomprehending and uncooperative. The family adviser can help the family to anticipate such difficulties. It is a good idea to discuss problems in advance with the family doctor, and, for dental care, to take the child for regular checks before any treatment is needed. The child can be prepared by playing games of 'doctors and nurses' and 'dentists' at home and in the nursery or school. As with all other experiences, a gradual introduction avoids many of the difficulties.

There are a few areas in which there is a dental clinic especially for handicapped children, or a dentist interested in this field visits schools and units for retarded children. Where special handicaps or difficult behaviour make it impossible for the child or adult to receive medical or dental care as an out-patient, it is sometimes possible to arrange for treatment to be carried out at the area mental-handicap hospital, using the services of visiting specialists.

Speech therapy and physiotherapy are ancillary medical services that are of special importance in the field of mental retardation.

Trained people are in short supply, and it is most economical of specialist time if the trained therapist teaches parents, nurses, and teachers to carry out the work under their supervision.

Help with practical problems

A mentally retarded person in the family can give rise to all kinds of practical problems including financial ones. Some of these can be alleviated by help from various central or local authorities or from voluntary bodies. The types of help available will be briefly mentioned here so that the family adviser can let the parents know what benefits they may be entitled to receive. Local authority social workers should be able to explain where and how to make appropriate applications.

A laundry service, free waterproof sheets, disposable pads, and plastic pants are obtainable through the local health authority in some areas. This is to help cope with incontinence in older children and adults. Wheel chairs can be obtained through the Department of Health. The local authority social service departments can arrange for special aids and adaptations to the home if these are required for the care of a handicapped person.

A 'baby-sitting' service for mentally retarded people of any age can allow parents to have an evening out together. Various voluntary agencies undertake this work and family advisers should be able to find out what is being done in their own area.

Parent groups may be run by workers in the local services or by voluntary bodies.

Social service departments can arrange for short-term care in hostels, residential homes, or hospitals to help in a particular crisis, to allow the rest of the family to have a holiday, or just to provide the parents with occasional relief from the strain of continual care. It is best to ask for this well in advance of the time when it is wanted, if such forethought is possible. Long-term care is also available, and will be mentioned in the next section.

There are a number of sources of financial help specifically for handicapped people and their families. The constant-attendance allowance is paid at two levels. The higher payment is made for people who need attention and care day and night, and the lower to those who need it only in the daytime.

A non-contributory invalidity pension is now payable to all disabled people over 16 years of age who are not at work. Those attending day training centres are eligible. For those receiving this pension, additional exceptional needs payments can be made for specific purposes such as replacing clothing.

The mobility allowance can be paid, in special cases, to people who are unable to walk more than 100 yards, but the rules for granting this are not yet clarified. There is also an invalid care allowance, again for special cases, where someone has to stay at home full-time to look after a handicapped person. This is not payable if the caring person is the mother, though it is to a father.

Applications for grants to cover particular needs can also be made to voluntary bodies concerned with handicapped people. One of the best known sources is the Rowntree Trust Family Fund, set up by the government but administered independently by the Joseph Rowntree Memorial Trust.

This list is not exhaustive, but does demonstrate that practical help is available if the effort is made to look for it. Such help can be invaluable in tiding families over crises, but too much reliance on outside sources may reduce the capacity to help oneself. A family adviser has to use all his judgement and experience in deciding what advice to give and how much to encourage the family to rely on 'the authorities'.

Organization of the environment

Although the eventual aim is to minimize behaviour problems by appropriate supervision, management, and teaching, it is sometimes necessary to organize the environment to prevent a mentally retarded person harming himself, other people, or causing damage to the home and its contents.

Running away loses its interest for a child if no one chases after him or shows any anxiety. Ignoring this behaviour is possible only if the child cannot run into danger, but this is rarely the case. If the problem cannot be dealt with in any other way, then doors to the outside should be fitted with special locks. Bolts or locks with catches that can be undone by hand are usually not effective, because a child intent on running away will soon learn to unfasten them and to find something to climb on to reach. Locks, of the kind made to deter burglars, which have to be opened with a key on both sides of the door are safest, as long as the keys are kept in a secure place out of the way of the child, or are carried by the responsible adults. Windows can be fitted with special fastenings to prevent opening, or to hold them open a few inches only.

Locks on internal doors to rooms and cupboards are also useful to prevent a child entering places in which he may do damage. If a child can play in the garden, it is wise to inspect the fences and the gate to make sure that he cannot wander out when unsupervised for a brief moment. It is surprising how quickly this can happen, even if a child does not usually move very fast.

Inside the house, cookers and heating appliances need to be guarded from children with no sense of danger. Electric points and electric wiring should be in good repair and safe from small hands. Matches and lighters of all kinds should be out of reach or, if necessary, locked away. If a child tends to break things, it is best to remove ornaments, crockery, and similar objects out of his reach as far as possible. Breaking windows may be a problem. If it is a frequent occurrence and the child persists in his destructiveness, unbreakable glass could be fitted.

Tearing wallpaper is a pastime much enjoyed by young children, and may last a long time in a retarded child. Some rooms can be kept locked, but the child's bedroom and the rooms in which he lives and plays can be decorated with washable paint instead of tearable wallpaper. If the child is not toilet trained and especially if he tends to smear when unsupervised, washable bedding, mattress covers, and flooring are all advisable.

If a child turns on taps and makes basins overflow thereby flooding the floor and perhaps spoiling furnishings, it may be helpful to remove the handles from the taps. This can be done by unscrewing some ordinary tap fittings. Otherwise, special taps with removable handles can be obtained.

In a house with a staircase, it may be necessary to fix a gate across the top of the stairs to prevent a child from falling. The handles on the rear doors of cars can be unscrewed to prevent them being opened when the car is in motion.

It is important to protect the retarded child and, as far as possible, prevent him from damaging the house and furniture. But the child is less likely to be difficult and destructive if he has suitable toys and a place, however small, where he can make a mess, pour water, tear up unwanted paper, scribble or paint on a large board or specially prepared piece of the wall, or occupy himself with any of the other activities beloved of small children. As always, a sensible compromise has to be found between the needs of the child and those of the rest of the family.

Financial assistance towards making a house safe for a handicapped person can be obtained through the local authority social service department, under the Chronically Sick and Disabled Persons Act (1971).

Long-term residential care

Residential care is necessary for almost all severely retarded people at some time in their lives. Most of those who survive their parents go into hospitals, homes or hostels, unless some other relative provides a home. When physical or behavioural problems are severe, parents usually find they cannot cope when their child reaches adolescence or early adult life.

The numbers of places in mental retardation hospitals are gradually being reduced. Residential homes and sheltered communities (for which local authorities pay fees for individual placements) are still being set up by voluntary and private bodies. In theory, if not in practice, local authorities should be increasing the numbers of places available in hostels within their own communities, so that mentally retarded people can remain within easy reach of their own homes, even when no longer living with their families.

Despite the present enthusiasm for care in hostels run on family lines, it is an unfortunate fact that adults who are aggressive, destructive, or who have other major behavioural difficulties, or severe physical handicaps, are very hard to manage in this type of residential home.

The aspects of care needed for such people are a high staff ratio, senior staff who are experienced in this type of work, close supervision and protection for those who may wander away or who are aggressive to others; plenty of space both indoors and outdoors; rooms where disturbed people can calm down away from other residents; and opportunities for simple physical activities such as walking or playing in water. In theory, such a service does not have to be staffed by people trained as doctors or nurses, nor does it have to fall within the definition of a hospital. In practice, it is rare to find such a protective environment outside the existing mental-retardation hospitals. Until alternative, effective services are set up, such hospitals will continue to be necessary.

When it appears that residential care may be necessary, the family adviser can help in two ways. First he can discuss the situation within the family and help the parents to make a reasonable decision in which the needs of all those involved are considered. Second, he can let the parents know about all the possible placements, and help them to make the necessary applications. As with other services that are in short supply, it is best if the possibility of care can be discussed well in advance, and the relevant authorities informed that the need may arise in the future.

When a place is found, the same gradual approach recommended before should be used. That is, the person concerned should, if at all possible, visit the hospital or hostel a few times before finally staying there. If the family can cope, weekends and holidays at home ease the pain of separation and preserve the place of the handicapped person in the family.

Final comments

In this chapter we have been mainly concerned with the problems rather than the rewards of caring for mentally retarded children and adults. This is a biased view, but inevitable in a brief article, because families seek advice when things go wrong, and not when they are progressing happily. To redress the balance a little, it should be said that some severely retarded people are the much-loved companions of elderly parents, and play their part by returning the love as well as giving a great deal of useful, practical help in domestic tasks. If such parents can be assured of a place for their son or daughter in a hostel, sheltered community, or hospital, with a comfortable, homely atmosphere when they themselves can no longer keep the home going, one of their main anxieties will have been relieved.

It should be clear from all the foregoing discussion that care for mentally retarded people within the community entails a network of supporting services throughout life. It is not easy for inexperienced people to find the help they require, since the available services are divided up among so many statutory and voluntary bodies. A family adviser who is knowledgeable about the area in which he works and who can guide families through all the complexities of the system is a valuable person indeed.

FURTHER READING

Baldwin, U. L., Fredericks, H. D. B. and Brodsy, G. (1973). *Isn't it time he outgrew this: a training program for parents of retarded children*. Charles C. Thomas, Springfield, Illinois.

Carr, J. (1979). *Teach me—I'm handicapped*. Penguin, Harmondsworth. [To be published]

Clarke, A. M. and Clarke, A. D. B. (Eds.) (1974). *Mental deficiency: the changing outlook*. (3rd edn). Methuen, London.

Finnie, N. R. (1968). *Handling the young cerebral palsied child at home*. Heinemann, London.

Hannam, C. (1975). *Parents and mentally handicapped children*. Penguin, Harmondsworth.

Jeffree, D. and McConkey, R. (1976). *Let me speak*. Souvenir Press, London.

—— *Let me play*. Souvenir Press, London.

Kiernan, C. C., Jordan, R. and Saunders, C. (1978). *Starting off*. Souvenir Press, London.

King, R. D., Raynes, N. V. and Tizard, J. (1971). *Patterns of residential care*. Routledge and Kegan Paul, London.

Kirman, B. and Birchnell, J. (1975). *Mental handicap*. Churchill, Livingstone, London.

Shearer, D. E., Billingsby, J., Frohman, S., Hilliard, J., Johnson, F. and Shearer, H. S. (1972). *The Portage guide to early education*. CESA, Portage, Wisconsin.
Tizard, J. (1964). *Community services for the mentally handicapped*. Oxford University Press, London.
— and Grad, J. C. (1961). *The mentally handicapped and their families*. Maudsley Monograph No. 7. Oxford University Press, London.
Wing, L. (1975). *Autistic children: a guide for parents*. Constable, London.
— (ED.) (1976). *Early childhood autism (2nd edn)*. Pergamon, Oxford.

7 Non-hospital residential care for adults with mental retardation

E. T. Udall and J. A. Corbett

Until the early part of the nineteenth century, with a few notable exceptions, the residential care of the mentally retarded and others suffering from chronic handicaps was undertaken to a limited extent by charitable or religious bodies. Mortality among the severely retarded was probably very high and for the more mildly handicapped who were unable to cope in the community, the only alternative was the public workhouse where they would have lived together with those unable, for other reasons, to support themselves in the community.

In mid-Victorian times separate institutions were developed by local authorities and this development was sanctioned by legislation which re-emphasized the need for custodial care. 'Mental deficiency' was associated with moral defect. Segregation protected society and the defective and prevented him from reproducing his own kind. Day care, although encouraged by the Wood report (1928), developed only very slowly and parents were often under pressure to send a retarded child into an institution from an early age. These institutions were usually sited far from the community they served and the resettlement of more mildly retarded adults with their families or in alternative residential care in the community was exceptional. It is only since the Second World War that the public have become aware that large numbers of mentally retarded people (some of them only mildly handicapped) are segregated in large, old institutions which are often overcrowded and understaffed. Several inquiries into allegations of ill-treatment of patients have highlighted conditions in some hospitals and brought pressure upon the policy-makers to speed up the allocation of resources to this sadly neglected field.

The Mental Health Act (1959) and the White Paper *Better services for the mentally handicapped* (1971) have changed the policy of care in large institutions towards the provision of smaller units in the community, from which residents can attend the same day centres that are provided for those still living at home with their families. Non-hospital residential care, however, has not been immune from criticism and fears have arisen that any precipitate or ill-planned move to smaller units may do little to improve the situation.

Most research in this field, particularly with the more severely handicapped, has focused on children. Tizard, reporting on the 'Brooklands' experiment, found that moderately and severely retarded children without severe additional handicaps cared for in 'child orientated' units showed a significant improvement in verbal ability and developed better emotional relationships and personal independence than children in hospital. Subsequent research by King, Raynes, and Tizard showed that local authority hostels were more child-orientated than hospitals, and that *effective* staff ratios (the degree to which staff spent time with children), the autonomy of the person in day-to-day charge of the unit, and the type of staff training, were the most important factors contributing to these differences. These factors were more important than actual staff ratios or the size of the units or the handicaps of the residents. The behaviour of the children, which may have been an important variable, was not measured in detail.

In planning residential services, decisions need to be made about the range of handicaps and ages of the residents who are to live together. The National Society for Mentally Handicapped Children has recognized the need for hospital provision for the 'grievously and multi-handicapped' individuals, particularly with behaviour problems, who cannot be coped with at home or in the informal unstructured environment of a hostel in the open community. The problem of behaviour disturbance in mentally retarded children has been dealt with in Chapter 6. In general, behavioural problems tend to diminish with age but they can remain severe during the teens and twenties and, together with physical disabilities, are then the chief determinants of the need for special residential and day care.

Miller and Gwynne, in a study of homes for the physically disabled, found that staff could build up defences against the pain and depression that such work entails. They suggest that institutionalism can be avoided if residents are involved in making decisions about the running of their own home. This may also help to safeguard them from disruptive alterations in hostel practices when staff change. Other studies of residential environments are discussed in Chapters 1 and 4.

Provision in hostels and group homes in England rose from 9.1 to 21.0 places per 100 000 population between 1969 and 1976; voluntary and private agencies accounted for about one-quarter of these places. In spite of this increase in numbers, at the beginning of 1976 hospitals still provided about 80 per cent of the total residential provision for retarded adults in England. Epidemiological studies have ascertained the prevalence of mental retardation in different areas of the country. The White Paper *Better services for the mentally handicapped* suggested that there are some 80 severely retarded adults per 100000 population living at home, and 150 per 100000 severely or mildly retarded adults in hospital or other forms of residential care. More recent figures suggest that relative and absolute prevalence figures can vary very widely between different areas. Thus, in 1970, Tynemouth was reported as having 24 retarded people per 100000 in hospital, while a comparable figure for Lincoln was 294. Population change can be a major factor and this is very evident in Greater London where inner boroughs have declined in population and outer-London boroughs expanded. At the end of 1970, Tower Hamlets, whose population had declined more than threefold in the previous 50 years, was responsible for 240 persons in hospital per 100000 while the figure for Bromley, whose population had more than doubled, was only 67. Before effective planning of a local community service can begin, knowledge of the numbers, characteristics, and whereabouts of the retarded people originating from the area is essential. This will need to be related to population change, social mobility, and changing patterns of handicap, and considerable caution needs to be exercised before extrapolating figures from other areas.

Characteristics of south London hostels.

In 1975 and 1976, the authors carried out a study of local authority and voluntary hostels for the adult mentally retarded in south London and the rest of this chapter is based upon the findings. The mobility, continence, and self-help skills of 219 long stay residents in 13 local authority hostels were assessed and a record was made of physical disabilities and behaviour disturbance. Similar information in less detail was obtained for 154 residents in 4 voluntary hostels.

There was a marked tendency to select less handicapped residents. In the local authority hostels only 5 per cent were over 60 years of age, none was blind, fewer than 1 per cent were deaf, and only 8 per cent had suffered from epilepsy during the previous year. Virtually all residents were fully mobile and only 1 per cent were severely incontinent. A number, however, had disturbed or difficult behaviour and wardens reported that 16 per cent posed severe management problems on account of behaviour.

A survey of all the adult mentally retarded in one area of south London (Camberwell), carried out by Wing and Hayhurst, provides data against which the degree of selection involved can be estimated. On the basis of current London practice, only about half of the Camberwell adults would be eligible for a place in a local-authority hostel. It is probable that hostels in other parts of the country also tend to exclude adults who are non-ambulant, incontinent, or have poor self-help skills.

Most hostels in the south London survey had fewer than 30 places. The staff–resident ratio on average was between 1:5 and 1:6. It was found that care staff usually had some responsibility for preparing meals but domestic staff were employed to do the main cleaning. There were no night staff, and care staff took it in turns to be on call.

This sort of staffing ratio means that in the smaller hostels (up to 15 places) only one member of care staff would be on duty. In two south London hostels there were only two care staff in all, they did all the cooking and had no relief for sickness or holidays. This is likely to affect the type of resident who will be admitted and restrict the activities of any resident who cannot go out unaccompanied by staff. In general, wardens of larger hostels of up to 20 to 30 places were more likely to accept a relatively wide range of handicap and ability than were wardens of smaller hostels. Effective resident–care staff ratios, the range of handicap and the size of the hostel are mutually interdependent factors.

Nine of the thirteen local authority hostel wardens in South London had a relevant qualification, usually nursing, while staff in smaller hostels were less likely to be qualified. One warden suggested that training might lead to discontent with domestic chores and with the salary, which would reflect the size of the hostel. King, Raynes, and Tizard suggested that staff with a nursing training tend to be more rigid than those with child-care training, but in South London the wardens with an RNMS training appeared to be more willing to take risks and to be more tolerant of disturbed behaviour, and in two of the hostels seemed to have gone out of their way to select difficult residents. They said they had left hospital, after a number of years experience of patients with difficult behaviour problems, to escape the rigidity and restrictions of life there, so perhaps they were exceptions. One can only speculate whether nursing training contributes to rigidity or whether it is merely a reaction to the hospital administrative structure.

Both the DHSS census in 1970 and the south London study showed that about half the residents in local authority hostels came from home, and about one-third from hospitals. Virtually no one was without weekday occupation and about three-quarters attended sheltered employment or a day centre, while one-fifth were in open employment. The DHSS census found that 46 per cent of residents required 'close supervision' without defining this. In south London, only 12 per cent of residents needed to go out escorted by staff, well over half the residents could go out alone. Physical incapacity, epilepsy, and past or present psychiatric illness restricted residents going out, and the severely retarded were considerably more restricted than the mildly retarded. The characteristics of individual residents did not account for the whole picture. Staff in the same hostel sometimes had different attitudes to letting people go out; and in a newly opened hostel, staff needed time to determine what residents were capable of, and perhaps overcome their own anxiety about allowing them out. Residents may need to get used to freedom of movement, or to the responsibility of accompanying less able residents.

Some wardens were more permissive than others; and this may affect the choice of residents. A nervous person may be better placed in a hostel with a protective warden than in a more permissive regime. The degree to which a person goes out alone, however, seems to be a reliable measure and useful in assessing social competence.

Restrictiveness and rigidity of routine may be dictated by practical considerations. The flexibility of mealtimes may depend on the availability of a cook, and a resident without a full sense of danger may not be allowed out alone. Any comparison between hostels must bear in mind differences in staffing and abilities of residents. In some south London hostels bedtime was fixed, in others flexible. In one hostel, residents were expected to bath daily, in others timing was usually optional with a minimum requirement of once or twice per week. Residents with single rooms could use them at any time. In some hostels, however, residents were discouraged from using shared rooms except for a particular purpose, e.g. changing, and sometimes there was some restriction on display of possessions, posters etc. However, in some hostels the accumulation of residents' possessions was becoming quite a problem on account of space. There were no formal visiting hours, but sometimes prior notification was encouraged; usually visitors could be invited to a meal. In most hostels, residents who were capable could make themselves a drink in the kitchen and in some hostels a snack also. Residents were encouraged to participate in hostel activities over and above their regular chores, and to help with meals, domestic work, gardening, care of pets, etc. In one hostel, with only two members of care staff, five of the twelve residents could go out only if accompanied by a staff member. Often the warden and a group of residents went on shopping expeditions or walked in the park.

This practice, which might be seen as 'block treatment', was dictated by circumstances.

Residents and staff usually appeared to relate together informally. In two hostels, staff on duty did not normally eat with residents, in other hostels, they did. There was no free access to staff accommodation.

Wardens usually felt well supported by the social services department, but there was a lot of criticism of field social workers on account of their lack of involvement, and ignorance about mental retardation and residential work. Perceptions of the role of the social worker differed and some clarification of roles and responsibilities seems necessary, particularly now that more residential staff are being trained. It was sometimes suggested that a liaison social worker might be useful.

There was much praise for GPs and no difficulty in obtaining medical services, but problems were experienced in getting psychiatric advice or inpatient treatment. Easy access to local psychiatric or mental retardation hospital services is essential; and instances were found of residents with psychiatric problems who had been admitted to the hostel before responsibility for their psychiatric oversight had been arranged.

In a few hostels, local retarded people were offered day or evening care or were invited to socials and outings; in all hostels residents could invite their friends. Wardens varied in the degree to which they were involved with residents who were moving on or had left. This depended upon the time and energy they had, and also on the amount of outside support available, e.g. from social workers, boarding out officers etc.

Some wardens felt that extra responsibilities might dilute staff efforts and depersonalize the hostel and that staff should concentrate on homemaking; the hostel was 'sacred to the residents' and any enlargement of its role might turn it into a less personal social services centre. On the other hand, some wardens felt that staff might welcome an expansion of their horizons from the rather inward-looking experience of hostel life, and that residents might benefit from offering as well as receiving a service. Contacts with the local community would be strengthened and local retarded people would get to know the hostel so that if admission became necessary, it would be easier for everyone. It would be useful if pilot hostels with some area responsibilities could be set up and evaluated.

The amount of contact with relatives was considerably greater than has been found in surveys of hospital patients but, even so, for nearly one-third of residents this was less than monthly. Generally, there seemed to be few informal personal contacts with other non-retarded people in the local community, although quite a variety of organized activities were available to residents. Some wardens had reservations about informal contacts; volunteers or befrienders were said to be unreliable, to have the wrong attitude to residents, to unsettle the residents, or to interfere with hostel management.

One of the most crucial aspects of hostel care is the range of activities and relationships that are available to residents and close contact with the local community seems to add an extra dimension to residents' lives. The development of such contacts needs initiative, time, and energy; volunteers need educating and supervising and can pose a threat to established hostel practices or the proprietal interest of staff in their residents. This is an area which should be thoroughly examined in staff training.

Hostel care should provide an environment in which a resident can have the security and care that he needs without unnecessary restriction or regimentation; bearing in mind the proper functioning of the unit. A generalization of this kind raises the question of how much restriction an individual needs, or how much his life should be structured. The hostel is the resident's home and staff are employed to enable him to have as satisfying and happy a life as possible. But staff will differ in their attitudes to their job and in their perceptions of what is best for the individual. However devoted, staff will have their own limitations which will affect practices in the hostel.

Staff will have differing ideas about what should be permissable, how much residents should conform to routine or particular standards of behaviour. In south London differing attitudes to homosexual activity in private were found, and some members of staff were more willing to allow residents to take risks than others. A warden has to reconcile and resolve different viewpoints among staff, and decisions will reflect particular viewpoints and ideologies. One warden saw herself as a mother figure who gradually allowed a resident to mature in a fairly protective atmosphere. Another warden was more inclined to push residents out into the world and allow them to find their feet. Both had their critics, but each did this job according to his own ideas. Until there is objective evidence to show that one approach is more valid than the other, criticism can be very destructive.

One warden spoke of his anxiety about allowing some of his rather disturbed residents out, and his ability to cope with this anxiety will influence the degree to which he will allow residents to take risks. Wardens have different personal standards, for instance with regard to sexual behaviour or personal hygiene. If a hostel is thought to be too permissive it is important to assess whether this is due to the inability of staff to curb excesses, or to a difference in viewpoint between the responsible authority and the care staff. Efforts to liberalize a regime may increase a warden's anxiety and thus decrease his ability to function.

The age, physical health, and stamina of staff will influence hostel practice. If it is considered a good thing that residents should go to bed when they wish, night staff should permit this. However, a staff member who has been on duty on her own all weekend and has prepared the meals as well may need to insist on a reasonably early bedtime. So too may someone who tires easily or has to unwind for an hour before going to bed. Staff numbers influence the situation; if two members are on duty one who is tired may be able to go to bed leaving the other to 'hold the fort'. Flexibility of routine will also depend on whether staff are resident or have to catch the last bus home, and the degree to which residents are able to take responsibility for themselves.

Staff vary in the degree to which they involve themselves in hostel life. In south London, the staff, to greater or lesser extent, separated work from their private life and restricted access to their own accommodation. One warden worked fourteen hours per day most days, others shorter hours. The time staff members spend in the hostel will depend not only on the staffing position but also on whether they are resident, and if married, the degree to which they (and spouse and children) are, or want to be, involved. One warden who had run a hostel for sixteen years said: 'When I'm off duty, I am off. I consider this a job of work.' Some people might criticize this attitude, on the other hand it has enabled her to give continuity to her residents over many years. Over half the wardens admitted to problems in separating their work from their private life. This was often due to the siting of staff accommodation within the hostel, with no private access.

Many factors of this kind give rise to differences of routine. It often seemed however, that where routine was organized to 'suit the staff' it was because it enabled them to cope with the job. In a utopian world, greater resources of staff and money might allow residents a much more satisfactory life, but perhaps the keynote of success in the real world is the mutual consideration of both staff and residents which implies a recognition of particular strengths and weaknesses of all the individuals concerned.

Aims and effectiveness

Residential provision may be long stay, rehabilitative, short stay, or a combination of these. In planning services, the degree to which a hostel can be selective must be decided and admission criteria defined accordingly. Lack of definition of aims may lead to some confusion of the role of the hostel and the sort of residents it should cater for, but too precise a definition, or failure to keep aims under review, may lead to inflexibility as needs change.

Aims are often expressed in general terms: 'to allow the maximum of responsible living', to offer a 'secure base', etc. Generalizations of this sort need to be translated into more specific policy goals. The south London study defined some goals which were felt to be important in preventing the formation of mini-institutions, namely the maximum personal and territorial autonomy for residents, their maximum involvement in decision making, maximum contact with relatives and people in the local community, and the maximum use of services for the non-retarded.

The perceived aims of a hostel may differ between the responsible authority and hostel staff. In south London, a number of wardens were not happy about the increasing long-term care function. One expressed concern about admitting the first person with Down's syndrome, another felt he had been appointed to a rehabilitative hostel which was now becoming a 'dumping ground' for the more severely retarded. Aims cannot be static and this should be borne in mind when engaging or training staff.

The search for measures to assess the effectiveness of a residential service is a difficult and hazardous process. The variables are many and complex and evalutation, unless it leads to improvement, is worthless. Much of the monitoring of hostel care must rely on the experience, sensitivity, and intuition of hostel staff and administrators, and sophisticated evaluation procedures, even if they can be worked out, may only confirm what is in fact already known.

In the south London hostels the only formal evaluation procedure appeared to be the case review, which was arranged in a few hostels. It is suggested that such reviews can be useful provided staff are motivated to hold them, and that residents, whether present or not, also see them as useful or, at least, do not resent them. Aims and policy goals for individual residents can be set and if findings are recorded using a systematic and standardized format, some measures of progress can be obtained, thus giving an idea of the efficacy of the hostel care.

Voluntary and private provision

Voluntary societies provide a wide range of accommodation for retarded adults. Hostels are run by religious orders and voluntary associations and some organizations place and supervise adults in foster and private residential homes. Although voluntary and local-authority hostels have many points in common, some differences were noted in the south London study.

The DHSS census in 1970 showed that, overall, voluntary hostels catered for some slightly less-able residents than did the local-authority hostels. This was also found in south London, but one factor here was the length of time some of the hostels had been open (in one case fifty years). Local authorities will also experience some deterioration in the abilities of residents as they age and this needs to be remembered in planning, for example, in the design of buildings. In 1970, voluntary hostels tended to be larger than local authority hostels and care-staff ratios slightly more favourable. In the South London study in 1975, only four voluntary homes were situated in the area. Three of these were relatively large homes with 63, 49, and 23 women residents respectively, and they were maintained by a religious order. A further small hostel with 25 places was run by a national society.

A number of adults with mental retardation originating from south London were placed in voluntary and private homes outside the London area. South London has a much greater proportion of people in such care than is found nationally; estimated in 1976 at 12 per 100 000, compared with 5.5 per 100 000 for England as a whole.

In the south London study the two larger voluntary homes had slightly less favourable care-staff ratios than the local authority hostels. The Order of Nuns which ran these hostels had provided care for many years, long before local-authority provision was available, and large buildings have been inherited from the past. Staff would have preferred a smaller unit, but whereas local authorities might have the resources to set up smaller units and then dispose of existing buildings, charitable organizations have not, and must adapt as best they can.

Staff in voluntary hostels in some ways had more responsibility than their local-authority colleagues. They were often responsible for upkeep of buildings, finance etc. and for continuous care. Greater responsibility, however, might be more widely spread; larger hostels employed a bursar and a housekeeper. On the other hand, care staff might be involved in weekday occupational activities. A comparison of staffing numbers is meaningless unless some information on their responsibilities is available.

Even if rates of pay are comparable, staff in voluntary hostels suffer some disadvantages. In days of inflation, pension schemes are less favourable, and secondment to training courses is less likely than in a local authority. These considerations were said to be serious disincentives to recruitment of staff. Advantages are less easy to identify and are inherent in the charitable and vocational nature of the work and the organizational differences between the two settings.

Residents in voluntary hostels are often sponsored by many local authorities, sometimes far distant. When crises arise or plans must be made, these authorities have to be contacted. Local statutory services may be reluctant to involve themselves with residents from another area, and it may be inappropriate for them to do so. This caused some problems, social workers were a long way away and demarcation difficulties sometimes arose with hospital psychiatric and mental retardation services. The appointment of a local authority liaison social worker might help and the availability of local psychiatric cover for all residents should be assured.

A resident from another area may not have access to local-authority training centres or social activities and, if he wishes to move into the local community, he may be at a disadvantage in terms of eligibility for sheltered accommodation or support. He may be doubly disadvantaged socially since contact with relatives may be difficult, but local voluntary associations may feel a particular responsibility towards people living in the local area and feel threatened by the impact of a large number of residents from the hostel. A resident who has lost contact with his home area, or who is wishing to move into the local community might sometimes appropriately become the responsibility of the local authority in which he now lives.

The whole future of voluntary services will depend upon the finance and support that is available from statutory bodies. It is to be hoped that they will co-operate to ensure that voluntary organizations are enabled to continue their work and offer opportunities and a quality of life at least as good as that available in local authority hostels.

In some areas, private hostels play quite a significant part in caring for retarded adults. Many retarded people from London live in such accommodation along the south-east coast. Here provisions may be expanding; hospitals have been under pressure to discharge patients and some private hostels have changed their function, finding that care of the retarded is less demanding than care of the elderly. No study of this provision seems to have been made. In the authors' experience it may range from good to very poor and in some cases day occupation is very inadequate. Local authorities have a very great responsibility, particularly if provision is far from the local area, to ensure that such people are not forgotten and regular visits are essential. Many residents may be more disadvantaged in terms of support and facilities than are residents in local authority or voluntary hostels.

A number of authorities, for instance in the London Borough of Croydon, have long had boarding-out officers and foster care is being developed in Solihull and other areas. It is difficult to find national statistics which is perhaps a positive sign as it means the retarded person is no longer someone whose movements must be recorded and quantified. This sort of care can provide a family or small-group setting for retarded people in his local area. It necessitates careful selection and education of foster parents and landladies, adequate support and day care facilities.

Group homes

In a local authority hostel the life of the resident is bound to be protected and restricted to some extent. A group home is likely to provide a more independent setting where the resident can develop in confidence and social skills. A social worker or someone from a hostel or training centre will need to give support and help with budgeting, homemaking, and interpersonal relationships, and a return to more sheltered accommodation must be available should the need arise. The group home may in turn be the stepping stone to completely independent living.

In Sweden this sort of care is well developed. Two hundred group homes were set up between 1970 and 1976, averaging seven persons in each home, and a further thirty homes were planned each year. Residents quickly developed the ability to make decisions and skills in home making and work attendance. This type of provision, although relatively inexpensive, is poorly developed in this country: yet in 1970 the DHSS census indicated that 25 per cent of adults in local authority hostels could cope in a more independent setting.

In advocating expansion of group home provision, we make the generally accepted assumption that a resident by assuming more responsibility, is thereby improving his quality of life. However, someone who has made a home for himself in a hostel may not wish to move on. He may have an important role in helping less-able colleagues and any dependence the hostel may create or reinforce may be outbalanced in terms of personality development by his contribution to the community.

The group home, however, is a necessary option in a community service and many residents at present living in local-authority hostels should be able to move on to this type of provision.

'The other half'

Existing types of residential provision in the community, if suitably expanded, could only cater for perhaps one-half of the retarded adult population and plans often seem to ignore the 'other half' whose only resort is hospital.

A striking finding of the south London study was the complete absence of non-ambulant people with mental retardation in the local authority hostels although some were found to be living in a voluntary hostel for spastics, most of whom were of normal intelligence. Others may have been living in hostels catering for the physically, as distinct from the mentally, handicapped. Under the age of fourteen, non-ambulant children, or those with severe difficulties in walking comprise one fifth of the retarded-child population, and 13 per cent of the Camberwell adult population in residential care were non-ambulant and living in hospitals. Many suffered from multihandicapping conditions, but about one-third, although non-ambulant and often dependent for self-care, appeared to be suitable for hostel care similar to that provided for the physically handicapped. Among these people was Joseph Deacon who wrote *Tongue tied* and whose life story has been featured on television.

'Joey's' life story illustrates some of the issues that arise when care of the physically handicapped, who are also labelled mentally retarded, is considered. He is an athethoid spastic with little useful function in his limbs and is confined to a wheelchair. He has a gross speech defect but good understanding of speech, and is dependent on others for all personal care. In hosptial he developed a close friendship with three other patients; two were ambulant and so could make their two friends mobile. The quartet between them produced Joey's life story. One interpreted Joey's speech, one wrote it down in longhand and the third typed it out.

In planning services, the views of the consumer should, as far as possible, be sought and taken into account. It is difficult to know how to determine the feelings and opinions of people who have difficulty in expressing themselves and the views of the more articulate may not represent those of the more retarded. Joey, however, speaks as someone who has lived most of his life in a large hospital. Life was what he made it and he and his friends made the most of the opportunities available to them. He does not comment on the size of the hospital, the building, the ward routine, or the lack of privacy, but there is not a page on which there are not references to his friends, relatives, staff, or voluntary visitors. The whole theme is of personal relationships and everyday occupational and leisure activities. He declares himself well satisfied with his life and his book would seem to indicate that the most crucial things for him are the nature of activities that are available and the opportunities for making relationships. Few people would advocate care in large institutions but hasty conclusions about their inappropriateness may be deceptive. Dogmatic statements about alternatives, unless based on good evidence or experience, may be detrimental.

If Joey had been born two generations later he might well have found himself in a hostel catering for the physically handicapped but his story raises a number of issues. What sort of provision should be planned for the more handicapped and retarded? Should they live in the community in groups with a wide range of ability and handicap, or with people who are similarly handicapped? What new opportunities can life in the community offer? Are we sure that by opening the door to a new set of opportunities we are not closing it on others?

Joey's label of mental retardation determined his future life. A considerable amount of work has been done in America to try and improve the validity of labels in mental retardation and assess their effect on the individual. Increasingly local authorities are being required to draw up registers of the physically handicapped and mentally retarded, and separate services are developing to meet the needs of these two catagories. In the health service, the individual tends to be directed to either the mental illness or the mental retardation service according to the label he has acquired—sometimes in the distant past. Labels create prejudice in the minds of both the labelled and the labellers and this tends to create barriers between services. Labels should be valid, constantly reviewed, and an asset rather than a liability. They should ensure access to the most appropriate services and not close doors to particular ones.

Joey's story, and many other instances in the south London study, show that residents living in a group with a wide range of ability and handicap can help each other and to some extent compensate for others' disabilities. A range of handicaps, however, can also pose problems. 'Dominance and servility' was mentioned by some wardens in South London and, particularly in small hostels, there were difficulties in arranging activities that would appeal to the community as a whole, or to a sufficient number of residents. The more able will be encouraged to arrange their own social life, the less able will need help with this. If hostels are graded by ability, this will create a hierarchy of units with the possibility of moving up or down the ladder. This may create a 'rat race' towards independence with feelings of shame if the ladder is not climbed or demotion is necessary. There may be advantages for the more dependent in a hostel with a wide range of handicap, but is this at the expense of the more able? How viable is a unit with a broad spectrum of ability and a diversity of aims both rehabilitative and compensatory? Questions of status and prejudice are involved, on the part of the residents, their relatives, staff and others and no simple answer is possible.

The size of the hostel is an important factor. The White Paper stipulates a maximum of twenty-five places for adults, but this has been criticized as much too large. In group homes a few residents live together. Minimally staffed hostels cater for perhaps ten or twelve able residents. The aim of a comprehensive service is to give the maximum benefit to the maximum number of people and the whole range of needs has to be considered. In Sweden, whereas group homes have an average of seven places, hostels for adults are much larger averaging 77 places but these are broken down into small living units. These hostels cater for some people more handicapped than their counterparts in England.

The south London study revealed a number of problems in small hostels catering for a wide group of handicap. The small hostel may be rather inflexible in a comprehensive service as it is likely to be more selective of its residents. For residents, there may well be considerable strain in living in a large group; but a small group may offer a very limited choice of relationships and activities. An answer could be found in providing each resident with a single room, in a small living group in a larger hostel. The larger total group provides a wider range of facilities, activities and relationships and may be more flexible because residents and staff can move between units if they wish or if particular circumstances, such as staff illness necessitate this. Once decisions have been made about the range of handicap that should be catered for in non-hospital provision, more research into the size of hostels, living units, and the range of handicaps seems necessary; and this in turn will determine the sort of building that will be best for the purpose.

In the south London local authority hostels the residents were mildly handicapped and a converted dwelling house was often very satisfactory and fitted naturally into the local housing of the area. This is seen by many as a great advantage but it is difficult to know objectively how valid this point is; and is possibly a subject on which residents' views could be sought. How much is the idea of a converted house a necessary step in the process of 'normalization' and how much a remnant of the idea that the mentally retarded should be hidden away, or a failure to accept that in some ways they are different? A converted house is likely to be cheaper, but one big advantage found in purpose-built hostels in South London was the much greater proportion of single rooms. However, hostels did not seem to have been designed with severely retarded residents in mind; one had been built on two floors above a training centre which precluded anyone non-ambulant. Purpose-built hostels should also be able to offer privacy and private access to staff accommodation, a point which was sometimes completely overlooked.

The concept of 'normalization' first originated in Scandinavia and may be seen as a reaction to the large hierarchical institution and a striving to achieve as near 'normality' as possible for each retarded person. Proponents suggest that residents should live in a bisexual world, in small group, with a room of their own. This idea was reiterated in the General Assembly of the United Nations resolution which declared the rights of the mentally retarded which stated: 'if care in an institution becomes necessary it should be provided in surroundings and circumstances as close as possible to those of normal life'. Such concepts must not obscure the fact that residential care away from home is not 'normal' and hostels and group homes constitute communities and not 'substitute family groups' as is suggested by the White Paper. The normal family group for an adult is with his spouse and children and this is denied to many retarded people, although staff may well afford residents care and affection similar to that of a parent. The concept of a hostel with the staff in the parent role does not recognize the adult status—at least in terms of age—of residents. Residential services should aim to provide an environment in which residents can be individuals with their own identity and the chance of optimum independence and self expression. Hopefully they will indentify with the community as a whole and be involved as far as possible in decision making. Within this framework they will need to experience satisfying relationships with other residents, relatives, friends, and members of the larger community outside. A logical corollary to the concept of 'normalization' would seem to be a recognition of a need for mutual consideration and concern about other residents and staff.

Defining responsibilities

In the White Paper the role of the hospital service is seen as 'treatment not residential care'. In the ideal community service long-term care in hospital will be necessary only if treatment is needed over long periods. There is a need for a definition of treatment, and hospital admission should occur only when treatment cannot be carried out on an out-patient or day-hospital basis. There are considerable variations in provision between different areas, and these are likely to continue until local authorities are obliged, rather than exhorted, to provide services, and until their responsibilities are more clearly defined. Lack of resources may delay expansion for some time, but now is the time to make decisions about *ultimate* responsibilities so that hospital and local authority services can plan together the sort of treatment facilities and residential accommodation that will be needed. Lack of such definition will only result in haphazard development and wasteful use of existing resources. For instance if larger hostels with small living units are eventually planned, then existing or planned hostels of 25 or 30 places may well become 'white elephants'. If many existing hostel residents move to more independent living, should not the buildings have been designed to allow some non-ambulant people to take their place?

Any transfer of responsibility is likely to be gradual. As a first step, it is suggested that local authorities should be obliged to assume responsibility for the sort of people catered for in most local authority hostels at the moment, i.e. those who are ambulant, continent, and able to manage much of their own self-care. Criteria for assessment may be difficult to define—particularly with regard to behaviour—but this is a problem also encountered with the elderly, mentally ill, and physically handicapped and is certainly not insuperable. There would not necessarily be a large expansion in hostel provision, since a number of more able people should be able to move on to group homes or boarding-out accommodation. A second step would be for local authorities to assume responsibility for non- and partially ambulant people who may need total help with self-care but are otherwise eligible for hostel care. There is evidence that this group is already being admitted to children's hostels. Severe incontinence at the moment is a major factor in excluding people from hostel care and decisions on incontinence are likely to be difficult and controversial. Resources devoted to research and training in an effort to reduce the size of the problem should be amply repaid in terms of quality of life for both residents and staff. Severe incontinence is invariably associated with other handicaps but the potential for training needs to be borne in mind and estimates regarding the size of the problem may be exaggerated due to poor staffing ratios in hospitals. There is also evidence to suggest that, as with behaviour problems, incontinence may be influenced by environment and is more marked in the barren environment of hospital than at home or in a hostel.

Alongside a policy regarding retarded people coming into residential care from home, there needs to be a policy about patients in long-stay hospitals. There would appear to be advantages if local authorities increasingly took over some responsibility for people in hospital. This might only be financial, but would encourage the development of alternative accommodation for those who wished to move back into the community, and progressive authorities would no longer be penalized compared to those who have provided much less.

There are many difficulties in planning for the future of patients in large hopitals, many of whom are elderly and some of whom, even if only mildly handicapped, may not want to move into the community. At the moment hospitals usually have the ultimate responsibility to provide care for those whom local authorities cannot or will not accommodate. They are often under pressure to reduce their beds, but cannot plan future services as they do not know if, or how, community services will expand. Local authorities, even if they had ambitious plans, have had to postpone them indefinitely. The provision for joint planning and financing announced by the DHSS is an encouraging step forward but until more concrete decisions are made as to the ultimate division of responsibility and the pattern of the future service, really effective forward planning is not possible.

Summary and conclusion

The adult mentally retarded who need residential care range from the able to the grievously multihandicapped. Before an effective comprehensive service can develop, it is necessary to define immediate and ultimate responsibilities as between local authority and hospital services, and these authorities should be obliged to meet their responsibilities. At the moment only the more able adults are catered for in non-hospital provision and local authorities have varying commitments and differ in the degree to which these are met. Much accommodation is in hostel-type accommodation although in some areas group homes, boarding out, and fostering schemes have developed. Eventually it is to be hoped that local authorities will have available directly, or through voluntary or private agencies, a series of such options within the local area and long-term hospital provision will be reserved only for those people requiring 'treatment' (suitably defined) which cannot be provided on an out-patient or day basis.

In considering hostel accommodation, the design of buildings, size of unit and staffing ratios will be influenced by the type and range of handicap that are catered for. The concept of 'normalization' suggests that a resident should have his own room and live in a small group, but this does not preclude the possibility of larger hostels broken down into small living units. Such an arrangement is likely to provide a wider choice of relationships, activities, and facilities and be more flexible in that it can be less selective and residents can, if necessary, move between living units. In hostels the needs of staff as well as residents must be considered; administrative constraints are real and the dynamics will be those of the community. Mutual consideration and an appreciation of the needs, strengths and weaknesses of each individual, whether resident or staff, are crucial.

Some restrictions and routine are inevitably present in a hostel. These may enable residents to develop, or staff to cope with their job. They should not be established just to make the task of staff easier. Many residents, however, are capable, should they wish, of moving on to more independent life. They may prefer to remain in the hostel and help their less able colleagues; this option should be available and if possible a 'rat race' to further independence should be avoided. The small minimally staffed hostel and the group home can, however, allow much more personal independence and enable residents to improve in self-confidence and social skills. Boarding out and fostering schemes can also greatly extend the series of choices and will provide accommodation that may be suitable for a wide varity of handicap and ability.

There is a wide range of possibilities. Development depends partly on resources of manpower and finance, but also on the initiative, enterprise, and enthusiasm of individuals, local authorities, and voluntary agencies. It depends upon policy decisions at the highest level and some authorities need clear guidelines about how to assess their own commitments, the changing pattern of handicap within their area, and the structure of the service they need to provide. More research may be necessary before such guidelines can be issued and a detailed study of countries in which services are more advanced would seem invaluable.

Planning of non-hospital residential care of the adult mentally retarded needs to take into account the total spectrum of needs. Decisions must be based on fact rather than on emotion and the individual should be allowed a choice of alternatives so that, as far as possible he can decide for himself which suits him best.

FURTHER READING

Baranyay, E. P. (1971). *The mentally handicapped adolescent*. Pergamon, Oxford.

Corbett, J. A. and Udall, T. *A home to go to: residential care for adults with mental handicap*. [In preparation.]

King, R., Raynes, N. and Tizard, J. A. (1971). *Patterns of residential care*. Routledge & Kegan Paul, London.

Miller, E. and Gwynne, G. (1972). *A life apart*. Tavistock Publications, London.

Tizard, J. (1964). *Community services for the mentally handicapped*. Oxford University Press, London.

8 Services for the elderly mentally infirm

Rolf Olsen

In terms of numbers and personal and social costs, the most urgent problem confronting our personal and medical services in the future is the care and provision of the elderly and particularly the elderly mentally infirm. This chapter begins by summarizing the changing age structure of the population and the likely trends in the number of persons aged over 65. It then describes the physical and social aspects of ageing, and sociological interpretations of these phenomena. The particular features of the elderly mentally infirm and the behavioural problems they present are also described. I then examine some assumptions about the efficacy of current hospital and other residential provision, before suggesting alternative strategies which might be pursued. The chapter concludes by examining the tasks and skills of the worker in the residential services for this group of people.

At the outset it should be stated that it is not always possible to distinguish clearly between the characteristics and needs of elderly people in general, and the elderly mentally infirm in particular. It would therefore be artificial, particularly when considering social and physical characteristics of ageing and strategies of care and prevention, to deal solely with the latter group as though there were no overlap.

The changing age structure

In the United Kingdom during the past 80 years the ratio of retired men and women in the population has increased significantly. In 1901, out of a total population of 38.2 million, 2.4 million, some 6 per cent, were of retiring age or over. By 1971 this ratio had changed dramatically; out of a population of 55.7 million, 9.1 million, some 16 per cent of the total population, had reached the official retiring age. Further, the average age of the elderly population is increasing rapidly. The DHSS forecasts that during the next 15 years the number of persons aged over 75 years will increase by 30 per cent, and the number over 85 years by 50 per cent. It is expected that the projected increase in the aged population will level off at the turn of the century, caused by the low birth rate of the 1920s and 1930s, only to return 10 years later to reflect the rise in the post-war birth rate and increasing longevity. Not until about the year 2030 can we expect to see the size of the aged population stabilizing.

A greater proportion of women than men reach retirement age and live significantly longer. Women account for three-fifths of all people aged 65 and over, and three-quarters of those aged 85 and over.

Physical and social aspects of ageing

When considering the physical and social aspects of ageing it is important to remember that a large number of the retired remain reasonably fit and active and economically independent for the greater part if not the whole of their reteirment. A recent survey of 2622 people aged 65 and over living in the community carried out by Audrey Hunt on behalf of the DHSS, showed that one-sixth of the men and one-twentieth of the women were working, and compared with evidence from other sources were likely to have as many hobbies and interests as younger people.

However, it is a fact that a significant minority suffer a considerable amount of physical, mental, and social hardship. Hunt found that loss of mobility, physical disabilities, and difficulty in looking after self increased sharply with age. (Five per cent of all elderly people are permanently bedfast or confined to the dwelling. The percentage rises from 2 per cent among those aged 65–74, to 20 per cent among those aged 85 and over. About one-fifth of the bedfast and housebound have not been outside their homes for over three years.) Personal tasks, such as cutting toenails, bathing, going out alone, using public transport, and undertaking domestic tasks which require muscular force and agility often require help to accomplish, otherwise they are left undone.

The elderly are prone to a wide variety of physical sickness and chronic illness, and present a special risk with regard to health. In particular they suffer from bronchitis, rheumatism, arthritis, anaemia, diabetes, and urinary-tract infections; they suffer a host of conditions associated with arterio-sclerosis; they are unsteady on their feet and therefore prone to fractures incurred in falls.

In addition to their physical disadvantages the old suffer considerable social handicap. They are amongst the most isolated and immobile. Two-thirds of elderly people have no help with their household tasks. Only 40 per cent possess a telephone and can use it without difficulty. Ten per cent never receive a visit from a relative, and 29 per cent of all elderly receive no visits from friends. Mark Abrams reported the results of a recent survey which showed that more than a million people aged over 75 live alone in acute loneliness of a kind which they had not experienced previously. Many have no remaining relatives and few visitors, and most reject any assoication with old people's clubs.

The elderly also figure prominently amongst the poor, and suffer greater poverty with increasing age. It is estimated that half of those over 65 live on or near the poverty line. In 1976 Hunt found that almost half the married couples had a combined income of less than £1500, and that 28 per cent of non-married women and 18 per cent of non-married men had total net incomes of less than £750 a year. Abrams reported that many of those he investigated suffered severe money worries. Two-fifths of those aged over 75 were unable to afford adequate heating and food.

In spite of this relative poverty, the elderly are reluctant to claim supplementary benefit. Atkinson (1969) found that almost 50 per cent of all retirement pensioners were entitled to claim income supplement, but that only half of those entitled to claim did so.

These disadvantages are compounded by the ignorance of the public about the needs of the elderly, the general disregard for their plight, and the comparitively low esteem accorded to the elderly. A recent survey showed that 63 per cent of the elderly have less than one contact per month with neighbours. Hunt found that one-quarter of her study group received no visits from a selected list of people from the health, social services, and voluntary agencies during the previous six months. These negative attitudes, which are due not only to our lack of knowledge and embarrassment about the physical, emotional, and social wants of the elderly, but also to a hangover from the sad traditions of the Poor Law, contrast sharply with the concern which is shown for the needs of children. Further, those professional persons who elect to work with the elderly rarely carry the prestige and status attributed to those working in other branches of medicine and social care. It is regrettable that in many social services departments the care of this group remains the least glamorous of the social worker's tasks, and it is one which is likely to be handed over to social work aides and the untralned worker.

On all fronts, therefore, it is probable that the elderly share with the mentally ill and retarded the lowest status, the least prestige, and the greatest public, political, and professional neglect.

Sociological aspects of ageing

The discussion so far suggests that for a significant number ageing can be a humiliating experience with little joy and few satisfactions. The evidence shows that this state is often determined by poverty, poor or inappropriate housing, social isolation, physical decline, lack of material resources and political and professional neglect. Brearley argues that many of the problems which face the elderly are due to structural features of society. For example, the emergence of the highly mobile nuclear family, and current house design which leaves parents isolated and unable to live with grown-up children; the pace of technical change which results in skill obsolescence and role loss; the speed of commercial developments such as decimalization and the increasing computerization of data, which causes confusion; and the rapid change in social values and attitudes towards behaviour, sexual relationships, debt, education, entertainment, etc. Unless the aged person is able continually to up-date his knowledge and make the considerable behavioural and attitudinal adjustments which are called for, this results in 'disengagement', manifesting itself in withdrawal and the avoidance of new situations which cause anxiety, and the maintenance of traditional and increasingly obsolete attitudes and ways of managing lives and relationships.

The characteristics of the mentally infirm

When considering the psychiatric problems which are found in the aged, it is important to distinguish between those conditions which are long-standing and remain into old age, and those associated with the ageing process. It is also essential to recognize that whilst senile dementia is the psychiatric condition usually associated with the elderly, they do, in fact suffer a wide range of psychiatric disorders. Five conditions stand out as deserving special consideration.

(i) Depressive states

Depression is a condition which increases in frequency with age. In such a state the person expresses feelings which range from mild gloom to utter misery and despair. He or she will complain of a variety of symptoms, depending upon the type and severity of the condition. These include difficulty in concentrating, an inability to cope with his affairs, loss of appetite, exhaustion, insomnia, and disturbed sleep. In more severe states the person is often self-deprecating, expresses ideas of guilt and blame, feels that life is not worth living, may be anxious and apprehensive, and may be a suicide risk.

Such states may be part of recurrent episodes which occur without apparent reason; they may occur as a reaction to an event which the person has found very distressing, such as bereavement or isolation and loneliness; or they may be consequent upon involutional changes associated with the middle and late years of life, and to such events as retirement, financial strain, physical illness, etc.

Depression in the elderly may be overlooked, or misdiagnosed as dementia because the person may become apathetic, unmotivated to do anything, or may be agitated and confused.

(ii) Confusional states

This term is used to describe conditions which are characterized by varying degrees of confusion, disorientation, memory failure, difficulty in concentrating, emotional liability, and inappropriate behaviour. Such conditions are often associated with physical illness of various kinds.

They may also be caused by the effects of drugs, particularly barbiturates, or be the result of disorientation caused by moving to strange surroundings or unfamiliar situations. A typical example of a confusional state is the elderly person who lives alone and appears to manage quite well until he or she suddenly wanders into the street at night dressed in nightclothes and causes a disturbance. On questioning the person does not recognize the inappropriateness of the behaviour, is confused as to its purpose, and is disoriented in time and place. It is important to recognize and treat any underlying physical illness.

(iii) Paranoid states

Paranoid states are characterized by a variety of unusual beliefs and attitudes of which the commonest is a feeling of persecution. This may range from a general suspicious and hostile attitude towards others, to a delusional state in which the individual believes that he is being adversely affected by events or persons which bear no relation to him. Persons with paranoid ideas are often fearful and secretive, and are reluctant to discuss their beliefs. This condition is not uncommon amongst those aged persons who are adversely affected by deafness and isolation and can accompany physical illenss or the early stages of dementia. In paranoid states personal isolation is often prominent due to the anxiety and hostility which is aroused in others.

(iv) Neurotic and personality difficulties

Neurotic and personality difficulties figure prominently in old age, often prove troublesome and make great demands upon those who live with and care for the elderly. It is thought that such problems are due to the difficulty in adjusting to and coping with changing and deteriorating physical, social, economic, occupational, and status positions of the elderly, at a time when people are less able to make a constructive psychological adjustment to adverse situations. The ever-diminishing world of the elderly, with no job, little money, isolation, physical ill-health, poor mobility, loss and death of friends, etc., results in the individual looking inwards, becoming increasingly egocentric, and expressing a continual morbid concern with unimportant events, relationships, moral position, bodily functions, and health. The result is that real and imagined difficulties may be exaggerated to a degree in which a proper perspective is lost, and activities and attitudes become circumscribed to meet the beliefs and values which are held.

(v) Senile dementia

Dementia figures largely amongst the elderly. It is estimated that 10 per cent of those aged over 65 have some degree of dementia. This percentage increases with age to affect 1 in 7 of those over 75 years. The condition has been described as the greatest generator of disability and dependence which affects physical, psychological, and social aspects of functioning.

In the aged, dementia is characterized by permanent impairment of functioning in which the psychological and behavioural changes associated with ageing are emphasized. The condition should be distinguished from the temporary confusional states that are commonly associated with illness or disease.

The major symptoms include memory failure, particularly of recent events; forgetfulness; reduced ability to concentrate; disorientation in time and place; an inability to make simple decisions; emotional lability; neglect of personal standards and hygiene; and hoarding.

Assessment of the degree and nature of the dementia is particularly important to ensure the most appropriate placement and pattern of care. Those persons with a mild degree of dementia and not suffering from significant physical disease or illness may be successfully managed at home, with appropriate support from domiciliary, day care, and social services. Equally, those with more severe dementia and showing a greater degree of confusion, restlessness, over-activity, noisiness, and incontinence can be cared for satisfactorily at home or in a residential home, providing there is appropriate support, particularly at night. If there is an associated physical illness which requires treatment in hospital, then admission to a medical, surgical, or geriatric ward should be arranged.

Present patterns of care

Notwithstanding the magnitude of the problems facing the elderly and their families, and the rapidly expanding aged population, at the present time we do not have the basis of a comprehensive pattern of care for the elderly infirm. Currently, 95 per cent of the aged live at home. A growing proportion of these suffer from severe mental and physical impairment and make huge demands upon their families, often with minimal or no support from the health and social services. In spite of this it is estimated that 95 per cent of the scarce resources allocated to services for this group are concentrated upon the hospital and residential services which care for 5 per cent of the aged population. There are many who believe that this is an appropriate distribution and argue that long-term if not permanent residential provision is the most sensible solution to this difficult problem. I hold a different view, and would like to argue that we must urgently reconsider the needs of the elderly in general and the psychogeriatric in particular, with the aim of radically changing our current patterns of care and distribution of resources. Before proposing the alternative systems which we might promote, I would like to briefly examine some of the assumptions about hospital and local authority residential care.

Hospital care

There is no doubt that in many districts the hospital services have developed a high standard of care which is sensitive to the needs of the mentally infirm and their families. Nor is there any question that a number of hospitals have pioneered major organizational changes, introduced important therapeutic techniques, and promoted a more enlightened public and professional attitude. However, it must also be acknowledged that hospital care has many disadvantages. It is the most expensive form of care, with each bed costing about £100 per week. Yet in spite of the high cost, hospital care with its appropriate emphasis on medical rather than social needs is often unpopular with staff, patients, and their relatives, and few regard it as the most appropriate way to offer long-term care. There is also evidence that hospital is not always the best place for the psychogeriatic patient, and that the medical knowledge and skills of hospital staff and the institutional regime is not conducive to the maintenance of social skills and personal mobility. In his discussion of geriatric care in hospitals, Whitehead wrote that to visit some wards for the elderly is to visit the annexe to the mortuary. He described rows of old people lying in bed, with legs bent and muscles wasted by lack of use, their eyes dull and vacant. They were old people waiting to die. Robb, in *Sans everything*, made similar criticisms, particularly of psychogeriatric wards. She found the treatment of senile patients caught up in a vicious system which resulted in understaffing, blocked beds, muddle, and overcrowding. Hard-pressed nursing staff, afraid of the consequences if a patient falls, are likely to conclude that it is better to confine a patient to bed or chair rather than risk a patient falling.

The raison d'être of a hospital and of the training and skills of their staffs clearly indicates that they must concentrate their efforts on the treatment and management of illnesses and other conditions associated with ageing, and not on offering a permanent resting place. An increasing number of geriatricians are giving shape to this belief by using their beds to provide short-term care or to accommodate 2–3 patients in rota.

Part III or local authority accommodation

Part III of the 1948 National Assistance Act allowed local authorities to provide residential accommodation. Although such provision remains scarce, in recent years a significantly large part of local authority budgets have been devoted to providing purpose-built accommodation and now little remains in the old workhouses. There are also signs that an increasing number of authorities are beginning to develop innovatory systems which emphasize the best principles of residential care. However, we are increasingly made aware that much of the new accommodation is unsatisfactory in a number of ways.

Great emphasis has rightly been laid upon the importance of building design in determining the model of care which is to be adopted. Design can create a living situation which offers residents a choice of how to spend their time, or it can effectively force them into a fixed pattern of life. Too often it is the latter. Thomas and his colleagues at Birmingham University have found during their researches into the provision of residential accommodation for the elderly mentally infirm, that confusion is often created in the elderly by badly designed buildings with endless corridors, complicated shapes and colours and repetitive elements.

However, even when purpose-built homes are designed along simple, uncomplicated lines, with easily-defined reference points, there is a great deal of evidence to show that such homes are not always satisfactory. In few instances do the residents 'make the rules', and as Mary Green has shown, 'Residents are often caught in the same bind as staff, a long day with not enough resources, a day that is formless and boring'. Even in homes with a high material quality we too often see the circle of tidy people, propped up in their chairs, without conversation or occupation.

Further, relationships between residents is often strained and unsatisfactory. In relation to psychogeriatric patients there is evidence that they are often unwelcome and thought to be unsuitable for this type of accommodation. Staff sometimes believe that they lack the skill and/or resources to care for this type of person, and alert residents are often intolerant of those who are confused and find their ruminations, rummagings, lack of hygiene, indescretions, and refusal to 'sit in their own chair' hard to bear.

Alternative patterns of care

In the foreseeable future it is anticipated that there will only be a marginal increase in the number of local authority and hospital beds available to the mentally infirm. However, this brief analysis has shown that even if there were a significant increase we would still be faced with the possibility that closed communities may not be the most effective way to meet the needs of the mentally infirm. Therefore we need to reassess our current methods of treatment and management, and to seek alternative ways of easing the handicaps and difficulties; in particular, ways of giving more support to relatives and to those who live alone.

The adverse consequences of current organization of services, methods of assessment, and models of care are numerous. In particular:

1. The assessment of individual and family need and the kind of help required is governed by the organizational framework and the methods used by the agency, not by the presenting problems.

2. The emphasis in diagnosis and care is on the individual client, rather than on his total social relationships and domestic setting.

3. This orientation leads to restricted help such as direct work with the individual client, and fails to consider the role and responsibility towards significant others, particularly the family.

4. The disciplines concerned with providing care tend to concentrate on old age as a *problem* rather than as a stage in life at which a

particular set of adjustments to health, income, leisure, changing roles, and employment are needed.

5. Lastly, the division between the services emphasizes their distinctions rather than the common purposes they ought to serve.

An alternative system for considering the professional tasks in meeting needs has been developed by Pincus and Minahan and Howard Goldstein. The model emphasizes that care should be concerned 'with the interaction between people and their social environment which affects their ability to accomplish their life's tasks, alleviate distress and realise their aspirations and values'. Therefore our services for the mentally infirm should have four main purposes:

1. To enhance the problem-solving and coping capacities of the persons concerned;

2. To link these persons with systems that provide them with resources, services, and opportunities;

3. To promote the effective and humane operation of these supporting systems; and

4. To contribute to the development and improvement of policy and organization of the services.

In assessing the needs of the psychogeriatric patient we must move away from the short-term, crisis perspective, and begin to focus on enriching the total life situation and the prevention of problems.

The mentally infirm: care versus rehabilitation

Central to this alternative model is the question of whether the mentally infirm can be rehabilitated. One traditional view holds that the primary need is for accommodation, and rejects the notion of rehabilitation. Many psychogeriatricians and others have shown this view to be wrong, and recent work, concentrated on the learning difficulties confronting the mentally retarded, and wondered whether learning difficulties of this group, has shown that it is possible to improve mental functioning.

For example, D. B. Lodge, Consultant Geriatrician at Carlton Hayes Hospital, observed that the deterioration of memory and understanding in the elderly was in many ways similar to the learning programmes used to educate the mentally retarded, could be used to improve the mental functioning of the confused elderly. He invited an educationalist, Frank Parker, to test this hypothesis. In his account which appeared in *The Times Educational Supplement* in 1974. Parker showed that 6 patients diagnosed as suffering from moderately severe senile dementia, 4 of whom were confined to a bed or chair, and all of whom were incontinent, were rehabilitated.

Essentially this technique, often known as 'Reality orientation' but sometimes called 'Resocialization and remotiveation', involves constantly reminding the patient of who he is, his relationship to others, where he is, the time and date, and always inviting his opinion in matters under consideration. Encouragement and praise are always used to reinforce self-initiated acts and independent actions.

In his final report on his study, Parker reported:

At the beginning all the patients were unresponsive, apathetic, perseverating and vacant. None was an individual person viewed from the door; all were a ward group. Some needed much help. In eight weeks mannerisms had minimised, folk looked to see who had come into the ward, they moved within the ward, incontinence did not exist. In twelve weeks all were said to be eating less, all had lost weight and were judged to be in better physical shape. In eighteen weeks occupations had been established about which some could converse. Greater recall was evident in all patients I talked with. At the end of the six months no patient had died. Chair-bound patients were moving voluntarily, self-help at meals was established, and an identity within the group and of the group plus its nurses—distinct from the rest of the community at social functions outside the hosptial—was well established.

The role of the social services

Community-based programmes.

The evidence clearly indicates that the primary aims of policies and social services for the elderly should be to enable them to continue as normal a life as possible and to avoid undue dependency upon relations, or admission to residential or hospital care. These aspirations mean that we must transcend professional boundaries and inspire new inter-professional initiatives which critically evaluate present care arrangements and promote systems of care which consider the needs of the individual within his total living experience. We must develop comprehensive preventative programmes which not only prepare people for stopping work but also for all the other personal and social adjustments which the individual will have to make. We require flexible retirement arrangements and policies which ensure that the aged receive an adequate income. The principles of commumity care must be underwritten by the provision of family care schemes; the wide distribution of clubs and day care facilities; the adaptation of houses which give attention to aids, and adaptation to baths, lavatories, heating, laundry facilities, safe floor finishes, alarm systems, etc.; the provision of home helps; *daily* meals on wheels; and the development of neighbourhood initiatives which aim to promote interest in the care of the elderly. The role of the volunteer must not only be recognized but actively supported and encouraged by the provision of resources which they require to achieve maximum impact.

It is only when these kinds of creative home support schemes and the provision of imaginative aids fail to meet stated needs that we should consider admitting an individual to residential care.

Residential care

If support in a residential setting is required, careful thought should be given to the possibility of placing in less restrictive environments such as sheltered housing and substitute family care.

Sheltered housing. The opportunity to possess a flat with one's own front door, which at the same time affords the opportunity to call for assistance when it is required, must represent one of the best hopes for a solution in the future. The scheme has the benefits of being relatively cheap, affording companionship and support, yet offering the chance of retaining privacy and independence. The arrangement does have the disadvantage of grouping the elderly together, and thereby running the risk of isolating residents and creating a geriatric ghetto.

Boarding out. To my mind this is a form of residential care to which we have given insufficient attention. The reasons for this neglect lie in the mistrust engendered by the scandals associated with the trade in lunacy during the eighteenth and nineteenth centuries, and by our disbelief in the motives of the entrepreneur who makes his profit out of caring for the mentally and physically frail.

Boarding-out is a descriptive term loosely applied to a number of arrangements with the common aim of placing a person in a living group to which he does not naturally belong. The schemes which I have investigated are operated in a variety of ways and differ significantly in terms of their size, the characteristics of the boarders, the type of residence, the care arrangements, the costs, and the clinical and social work supervision and support.

The overall conclusion one must reach about the opposing views as to the value of boarding out in the management of persons with psychiatric and psychogeriatric disorder is that they are speculative, largely based on opinion, beliefs, and clinical or social work experience. To date, no properly controlled and validated investigation, or a comparative analysis with other forms of care has been attempted. However, it is important to note that the studies which I have seen suggest that the strategy may be of value, and that it could form an important part in the spectrum of care for the psychogeriatric patient.

For example, Gertrude Smith in 1975 reported the results of a project in which in one year she found homes with families for over one hundred long-stay patients discharged from psychiatric hospital. The majority of the 105 patients in the study were over 60 years of age, some over 70 years, and the oldest 88 years. None were considered able to look after themselves in supervised flats or group homes. At follow-up over one year later, only 3 had died—all over 80 years of age— and none had been readmitted.

Following my own research into the success of boarding out the long-stay psychiatric patient, I concluded that with important reservations, these residences were successful and that they offered a viable alternative which had many advantages over hospital and local-authority provision. In particular they enabled patients to live within the community, offered a high standard of care, a greater degree of independence, the opportunity for self-determining behaviour, and the chance of an increased dignity from the possibility to contribute to the well-being of others.

However, it is important to acknowledge that perhaps the majority of boarding-houses, as they are at present operated, primarily serve as holding environments, in which there is a low expectation of achievement and initiative. The result is that when we place a person in a boarding-house we locate them in miniature institutions, which does little to circumvent chronicity or achieve rehabilitation.

The blame for this must lie in the exploitation of landladies and their residents and in the failure of a number of hospital, local authority, and other services to support the venture. It is a sad reflection that 20 years after Wing's report of the family care systems in Norway and Holland, the care and support given to boarding-houses in this country completely fails to match the standard which he reported. If we are to utilize this valuable community resource to the full, then we must give a fair financial payment to ensure that the landlady receives a proper return, is able to employ help and avoid overcrowding; particular attention must be given to the selection of patients and ways devised to try to reduce the behavioural and care problems which they present—particularly in relation to the neglect of hygiene reported by the majority of the (83 per cent) landladies in my study; the educational, social, and occupational needs of the residents require careful evaluation and the provision of an appropriate range of recreational, occupational, sheltered workshops and day centre services; the house must receive continuing support from the medical and social work services;

and efforts should be made to promote community acceptance of the houses and integrate the patient into the community. It is only by these efforts and the application of these resources that we will avoid relocating the patient in a sheltered sub-society, stop regarding boarding-houses as a side-line undeserving of our attention, and begin to develop the full potential of this primary resource.

General principles and values of residential care

1. *Purpose*. Residential care should not be seen as the final solution but as a significant cog in the wheel of total provision. It should be regarded as part of the total community resource, and aim to involve the community and other services in its activities.

2. *Total needs*. The emphasis in care should always be on the total needs of the individual. This includes a concern for the emotional, physical, social, educational recreational, and occupational needs.

3. *Privacy and independence*. The right to privacy and independence should be acknowledged and opportunities provided to enable the individual to reduce dependence, to state individual preference, and to excercise choice.

4. *Shared goals*. Good residential care involves collaboration between staff and residents in establishing capacities and needs, determining goals, and agreeing the strategies to achieve them. The 'contract' should clarify needs and the alternative goals, as well as the resources available to achieve them.

5. *Treatment and management*. Too often the treatment focus is narrow, and is one which emphasizes the alleviation of problems rather than a concern with total functioning and enrichment.

6. *Maintenance of outside contacts*. Attempts to contain the residents exclusively within the institution should be resisted. All residents should be actively encouraged not only to maintain established contacts with relatives and others outside the residence, but to develop new associations with individuals and groups.

7. *Participation in organizations*. In the belief that maximum happiness and progress is likely to be achieved where there are opportunities for reciprocal relationships, it is essential that residents are involved in the organization of the residence and in determining the rules which govern.

8. *Physical structure*. The importance of good design and decoration for this client group has already been discussed.

General tasks and skills required

The model of care to be adopted, together with the tasks and skills required to fulfill the objectives, should be clearly understood and agreed by the staff. The CCETSW discussion document *A new pattern of training for residential social work* identifies and outlines the major tasks and skills of the residential worker. In particular it emphasizes the importance of:

(i) Tasks

1. *Participation in decision to admit into residential care.* In line with the principle of shared goals, residential workers and clients should be jointly involved in decisions regarding the most appropriate treatment to be offered and whether to admit the client into residential care.

2. *Admission to residential care.* The process of admitting the mentally infirm into residential care should be designed to create the maximum participation and minumum disruption and distress to the individual and the relatives. The process should convey that the admission is part of a planned programme and not a last resort.

3. *Establishment of goals and development of a care programme.* These should be interprofessionally designed, not only in terms of the needs of the individual resident but also according to the needs of the total residential group, the relatives and all significant others.

4. *Regular review.* The identified goals, related to each person and the systems and groups to which he belongs, should be regularly reviewed in terms of how far they are being achieved and their continued appropriateness.

5. *Community support.* Action should be taken to encourage community and volunteer support and participation in the goals and strategies of the centre. The care of the mentally infirm requires a high staff—client ratio but this is rarely if ever available. Pairing a volunteer with a resident and his family in order to befriend and take a particular interest can help to overcome this shortage.

6. *Discharge.* The planning for discharge and the provision of alternative services once the goals of residential care have been achieved must be carefully undertaken.

(ii) Skills

To fulfill these tasks the residential worker needs to develop skills not only in working with the individual but also with the different systems to which his clients belong—natural living groups, social groups, the community, etc.—as well as with others who have a professional concern. This requires the ability: to establish close working relationships with individuals and groups; to diagnose problems and clarify needs; to determine alternative goals and the strategies to achieve them; to undertake agreed strategies and employ the skills required to promote the desired changes; to stabilize the change once it has been achieved; and, if appropriate, to arrange return to the community and to refer to other agencies once the goals have been achieved. Of course a primary skill in the residential care of the aged and mentally infirm is the ability to relieve suffering, to give comfort, and preserve the dignity of those who are dying.

To these tasks can be added the skills required to work with the residential group itself, not only to resolve its difficulties but also to promote the benefits of group living and mutual support. The CCETSW Discussion Paper defines (page 18) the skills involved in working with groups in residential settings as: understanding the nature of interaction within the group; helping it to mobilize its own resources; creating opportunities for leadership amongst the members; helping to minimize the destructive elements and to resolve conflict; and promoting the toleration of differences.

Rules and regulations form a part of all institutional living, but they should be kept to the minimum, formulated in discussion with all the residents, and reviewed regularly. The provision of care and clothing, the serving of food and the allocation of living space should be done in such a way as to ensure that choice is exercised, dignity maintained, and individuality preserved.

(iii) Specific tasks and skills

In considering the psychiatric care of the elderly mentally infirm, perhaps the major problem to be overcome is the mistaken belief that all disturbed elderly people suffer from dementia and are not subject to the variety of disorders described earlier. The result is that the disturbed behaviour of many elderly people is misdiagnosed, deafness is interpreted as confusion, and poor sight as lack of interest. This belief often leads to the view that there is little scope for therapeutic intervention, and that the major task of the care staff is a caretaking role. If this view prevails it results in a care situation in which the primary aim of the staff is to 'contain' the *patient* and to prevent wandering, injury, and unacceptable behaviour, etc. In consequence doors are locked, false teeth and personal possessions are put away, and the *person* is kept in bed or chair-bound for long hours. Unless it is recognized that all persons with mental disorder, irrespective of age, require careful diagnosis and should be given the treatment and care appropriate to the condition and the individual need, then the client is severely disadvantaged and the purpose of the residential unit reduced to a custodial role.

In general the initial psychiatric care consists of managing the immediate or presenting symptoms and in making efforts to establish a good relationship with the person. This allows for a period of careful observation in which a diagnosis and long-term treatment and management is decided. In reaching these decisions team-work between the residential workers, doctors, field social workers, nurses, psychologists, and all other professionals involved in the case is essential. It is also most important to establish a rapport with the person and his relatives which is based upon mutual trust and respect and upon a genuine exchange of ideas.

The overall role of the residential worker in relieving mental infirmity should be governed by the aspiration to rehabilitate. The specific roles should be dictated by the particular condition suffered by the individual. In some conditions such as depression and confusional states, the major treatment will be appropriate medication and other physical treatments. In paranoid states, neurotic and personality disorders, and in senile dementia, the residential worker will have a larger role to play. Often the most important and perhaps most difficult role with persons with paranoid ideas is to persuade them to regularly take prescribed medication which is necessary to keep the symptoms within tolerable limits. It is also important to try to lessen the isolation and the hostility and anxiety which paranoid persons arouse in others. Most important is the relationship between the person and those who care for him. The care staff must not argue with the client about his delusions but make it clear that whilst they understand the beliefs and the anxiety which they cause, they do not share or subscribe to them.

The management of neurotic and personality difficulties in the aged present particular problems to the care staff, not least because the elderly often find it difficult to give up the seemingly entrenched values, ideas, or beliefs which they hold. However, there are a variety of techniques which can be considered and appropriately used, based upon group work, behaviour therapy, and psychotherapy. These methods aim to bring about changes in personality, anxieties, behaviour, and understanding by modifying behaviour and response or by increasing the individual's understanding of self. The techniques may be specifically employed in treatment sessions or built into the ongoing situation. For example the use of 'reality reinforcement' will contain techniques of behaviour therapy; the principles underpinning the discussed values, tasks, and skills may reflect the style of casework or psychotherapy; and work with the whole group requires skills in group work.

The specific roles of the residential worker in relieving senile dementia were discussed earlier. To manage successfully the associated problems of immobility, passivity, disinterest, boredom, and withdrawal, the care staff must ensure that they constantly involve the client in all that is happening in the environment. This calls for much encouragement, the maintenance of the individuality of the client, and the promotion of independent behaviour. This means not only ensuring that the person undertakes responsibility, as far as is possible, for toilet, dressing, care of belongings, etc., but also has the opportunity to state individual wants and preferences which are respected and acted upon, and that each day is appropriately and purposefully occupied.

The care staff must also ensure that neglected physical disabilities are not compounding the problems associated with the mental disorder. For example, it is important that hearing aids are not only provided but are also in working order, dentures must fit correctly, eyesight must be regularly assessed and spectacles checked and kept clean, and aids should be provided wherever necessary to promote movement and independence. It is also important to ensure that clothes and shoes are the person's own choice and are clean and well fitting.

It is only by a concern with the integrity and well-being of the individual, the rejection of the custodial role and the promotion of the therapeutic environment that it will be possible to surmount the disadvantages associated with the residential and institutional care of the mentally infirm.

FURTHER READING

Abrams, M. (1978). *Beyond three score years and ten*. Age Concern, London.
Atkinson, A. B. (1969). *Poverty in Britain: the reform of social security*. Cambridge University Department of Applied Economics: Occasional Paper No. 18.
Brearley, P. (1976). Social gerontology and social work. *Br. J. Social Work* **6**, 443.
CCETSW (1974). *Social work: residential work as part of social work*. CCETSW Paper No. 3.
DHSS (1972). *Services for mental illness related to old age*. HMSO, London.
— (1975). *Better services for the mentally ill*. Cmnd. 6233. HMSO, London.
Goldstein, H. (1973). *Social work practice: a unitary approach*. University of South Carolina Press, Columbia.
Green, M. (1977). Aspects of old age. *Br. J. Social work* **3**, 301–20.
Hunt, A. (1978). *The elderly at home*. HMSO, London.

Olsen, M. R. (1976). Boarding-out the long-stay psychiatric patient. In *Differential approaches in social work with the mentally disordered*. BASW, 16 Kent Street, Birmingham B5 6RD.

Parker, F. (1974). Second childhood. *Times Educational Supplement*, August.

Robb, B. (1967). *Sans everything*. Nelson, London.

Smith, G. (1973). Institutional dependence is reversible. *Social Work Today* **14**, 426–8.

Thomas, N. (1977). Research into the provision of residential accommodation for the mentally infirm. Birmingham University.

Whitehead, A. (1970). *In the service of old age*. Penguin, Harmondsworth.

Wing, J. K. (1957). Family care systems in Norway and Holland. *Lancet* **ii**, 884–6.

9 Principles of the new community care

J. K. Wing and Rolf Olsen

In this chapter we shall attempt to bring together the suggestions made, on the basis of their empirical studies, by the contributors to this volume. Up to the 1950s, the centre of care for severe and chronic psychiatric disability was the large psychiatric hospital, though there were subsidiary centres in the out-patient departments of general hospitals and in local authority medical or welfare departments. Much of the movement towards a radical restructuring of services originated in these hospitals and was reflected in the discharge of long-stay patients; the decreasing length of stay of newly admitted patients; the creation of new centres of care outside hospital as psychiatrists, nurses, occupational therapists, teachers, and social workers saw new kinds of opportunity for helping disabled people; and the shift of emphasis towards primary forms of care by general practitioners and social workers with the intention of preventing illness and disability.

It is generally agreed that these trends have been in the right direction but that the new ideas which have been applied in all three major areas of psychiatric disability (mental 'illness', retardation, and infirmity), have not yet been thoroughly verified and tested, either in theory or in practice. The health and social services have not developed in balance with each other, the theories of doctors and social workers have seemed to be conflicting, and the views of consumers (particularly the handicapped and their immediate relatives) have not been taken sufficiently into account. These problems were not caused by a shortage of money for building new forms of service but they were greatly aggravated by it. In 1973–4, for example, £300 million was spent on hospital services for the mentally ill compared with only £15 million on personal social services (£6.5 million of it on residential and day care). Expenditure on residential after-care services for the mentally ill accounted for only 0.04 per cent of all local authority spending.

The White Paper of 1975 was nevertheless unduly pessimistic: 'Delay in building up local services must mean too that it is unlikely that we shall be able to see in every part of the country the kind of service we would ideally like within even a 25-year planning horizon.'

The build-up of NHS non-residential services, including local out-patient departments, day hospitals, rehabilitation workshops, domiciliary visiting, community nurses, and general-practitioner care means that an increasing share of the health budget will be devoted to functions that overlap with those of the social services. The use of hospital–hostels points in the same direction. Voluntary services have also been building up rapidly, using public funds in a new way: sickness and disability benefits, housing associations, provision for homeless persons, subsidized rents in boarding-out schemes, and so on. Group homes have proved cheaper than hostels and often quite as effective. There are many other innovations in store, particularly if new ways can be found to link and plan medical and social services together.

We are not attempting, in this chapter, to present a blueprint for an ideal service since we do not think that any one blueprint will suit the needs of all areas. The principles of community care can effectively be embodied in many different patterns of service. We are concerned with the principles themselves, some of which are now well enough understood to be generally agreed, others of which are still obscure or controversial.

Interaction between clinical and social problems

Perhaps the most fundamental principle is that there is always an interaction between clinical and social problems. It is rarely possible to separate the two in a way that would be convenient for the development of independent medical and social services. Social behaviour is affected in different ways by acute or chronic psychosis (Chapter 2), by language impairment and intellectual retardation (Chapter 6), or by progressive dementia (Chapter 8), but, in each case, it is not only the handicapped individual who has to cope. His or her family, neighbours, employers, workmates, and professional helpers, as well as society at large, are involved. On the one hand, there are the specifics of impairment: the delusions and hallucinations, the slowness and underactivity, the inability to understand social rules, the poor memory. On the other hand, social factors can exacerbate or ameliorate impairment, contribute to adverse personal reactions or to a positive use of talents, and affect the coping ability not only of the disabled individual but of all the other people involved with him or her.

We know that a socially intrusive environment, whether in a ward, a rehabilitation unit or at home, can lead to relapse in schizophrenia (Chapter 2). This is most evident in family studies but the principle holds good for all social environments. The same is true of social understimulation which leads to an increase in the 'clinical poverty syndrome' (Chapter 1). The interaction is most evident in large, understaffed wards but it can occur in a group home. A child who has not developed the ability to use language-related skills up to the level of his non-verbal ability will tend to become severely disturbed in behaviour unless those looking after him recognize his problems and help him cope with them (Chapter 6). The principles according to which help needs to be given are the same whether the setting is a ward, a residential school, a hostel, or the family. An elderly person whose memory is imperfect, who has difficulty in recognizing others and in finding her way about, will experience much more severe disability in unstructured and unfamiliar environments, whereas a familiar routine with plenty of clues as to identity and orientation will minimize impairment (Chapter 8). Again, the principle holds true across social environments.

The ability to recognize the main types of impairment present, and what social factors are likely to make them better or worse, is part of the knowledge that relatives, professional helpers of all kinds, and (so far as possible) disabled people themselves, need, in various degrees, to acquire. A different kind of knowledge, with different implications, is that concerning deprivation or social disadvantage. The distinction between impairment and disadvantage is particularly clear in tracing the origins of destitution (Chapter 5). Most people who were severely deprived as children do not become destitute, nor do most people who develop severe mental impairments, but the combination of disadvantage and impairment is deadly. To a lesser degree, many people who accumulate in sheltered settings such as group homes and day centres are both disadvantaged and impaired. It is important to realize, therefore, that different techniques of compensation and prevention are needed and that sometimes the methods that seem appropriate for one type (e.g. experience in getting used to the pressures of competitive employment, which might be very helpful to someone who has not previously had an opportunity to acquire it) may actually be harmful for the other (e.g. if someone with schizophrenia has broken down under just such pressure). Developing social and occupational and domestic skills and talents, so as to make the working day more profitable and leisure time more enjoyable must go hand in hand with a recognition of how much it is reasonable to expect a disabled person to achieve.

The other type of factor contributing to disablement, the development of adverse personal reactions such as undue dependency, institutionalism, low self-esteem and under-confidence, is a response to the experience of impairment and disadvantage (and to other people's attitudes to these problems). Reducing impairment and disadvantage should therefore diminish secondary reactions also. Once dependency or under-confidence has developed, however, it acquires a persistence of its own and can be very difficult to correct. It can therefore happen that severe social disablement is due entirely to such secondary factors, when impairment is minimal and social disadvantage correctable, and the major problem is that the individual has no confidence in an ability to function adequately which those trying to help him know he, in fact, possesses. This is where peer-group pressures, and individual support from a trusted counsellor or friend, can often prove decisive.

Social disablement is usually due to a combination of these three elements but, at any given time, one component is often more responsive to ameliorative action than the others. Recognizing the elements, and providing the right help in the right social environment at the right time is not purely a matter of common sense. It requires training and experience of a breadth that will not be available while training courses are based on professional disciplines rather than on the problems of disabled people and their families.

Components of care

We have used the term 'care' very broadly, to include treatment, rehabilitation, counsel, support, shelter, and welfare. It is not within the scope of this book to discuss these concepts in detail but we are concerned with the various ways in which acute illness, chronic impairment, social disadvantage, and adverse personal reaction can be prevented, or minimized and then maintained at the lowest possible level. In the course of long-term disablement all these components are likely to be experienced in various combinations. It may be convenient for care-givers to specialize in the provision of one or other type of help but unless each is at least aware of the range of possible needs and unless there is provision for an overall assessment up-dated at regular intervals, there will be no possibility of continuity.

'Treatment' should be used strictly to refer to methods of decreasing the severity of symptoms. Social methods of treatment are fully as important as physical means such as medication. Some examples have been given in the preceding section.

The concept of rehabilitation has been discussed in Chapters 1 and 4. As the principles of continuous 'management' become widely accepted and applied throughout a network of co-ordinated sociomedical services, most of the occasions for spectacular 'successes' (of the kind that used to be seen when new methods were being introduced to psychiatric hospitals) will disappear. 'Rehabilitation' implies the restoration of a previous level of functioning. The term 'resettlement' rubs home this idea. In fact, to adopt such an aim, when impairments are severe and long-lasting, is to invite failure. What handicapped people need is experience of success. The experience described in Chapters 1, 4, and 5, suggests that increasing the number of options available is the appropriate model to use. This will enable people with different kinds of difficulty to advance at their own pace and to achieve a permanent settlement at the level of minimum disability. If the highest level achievable is living within a sheltered environment, achieving this level is a form of success and not a form of failure.

Perhaps the classical model of 'rehabilitation' is most applicable to the correction of social disadvantages (when the severity of impairments allows this). Education and training for occupational and domestic roles, as well as for self-expression and fulfilment, is an obvious example of increasing the options.

This useful concept of rehabilitation should not displace the equally useful concept of 'maintenance'. Quite often, what is required is to keep up a level of social activity (including elements of occupation, self-care, and social interaction); the standards of success being the maintenance of a stable but limited improvement, because this means that deterioration is being prevented. The reward to the care-giver is the knowledge that, but for the provision of these opportunities, social disablement would be very much greater. It takes considerable experience to appreciate when a maintenance, rather than a rehabilitative, aim is best pursued.

Terms like 'resocialization' carry a similar connotation to 'rehabilitation'. They can be used in an exact sense (i.e. to restore function to someone who has been 'desocialized') but some people have impairments that prevent their being very sociable, and what they need is to find a way of living in which this impairment is least disabling. Moreover, 'desocialization' is often a misnomer for socialization of a 'deviant' kind such as takes place, for example, in drinking schools. Archard has pointed out that destitute men belonging to such schools, far from being desocialized, adopt strict social conventions dictated by their need to obtain daily supplies of alcohol and to keep out of trouble so far as possible in their public way of life. Unrecognized moral assumptions are often involved in the adoption of terms such as 'desocialization' and an element of impairment is often implicitly denied.

The concept of 'living with' psychiatric disability is one that has not yet been sufficiently explored. It has implications for the disabled person, for the relatives, and for professional helpers. We may take schizophrenia by way of example. There may be a long history of social disadvantage before the first episode of florid symptoms, which is followed by repeated relapses, with severe chronic impairments (slowness, apathy, social withdrawal, thought disorder) accumulating in between, and complicated by an understandable unwillingness on the part of the disabled individual to believe (in spite of definite talents) that there is any chance of living a life of any achievement. In fact, many important factors lie in the hands of the disabled person, some others in the hands of relatives, and some in the hands of helpers. The problem is to manage all these factors so as to promote an optimum settlement. Professional people have failed to capitalize on the potential capacity of disabled persons and relatives, helped by skilled counselling and support and the use, when necessary, of various kinds of specialized social environments, to acquire considerable skill in living with disability. With the emergence of voluntary bodies representing people with various kinds of disability, there is now an opportunity to put right this neglect. Diana Priestly describes one promising experiment which could provide a model for other areas.

The concept of 'shelter' also needs reappraisal. It includes that of 'refuge' or 'asylum' and that of 'protection'. Sometimes, all that is needed by a person who has broken down under stress is a quiet place in which to recuperate. Sometimes, impairments are so severe that the individual is permanently in need of care throughout most aspects of living. In such a case, protected domestic and occupational environments are required and a private outdoor space as well. Most often, the need for shelter is partial—for example, in the sphere of occupation, or of self-care, or of social amenities, only. When relatives provide this protection a common preoccupation (particularly among parents) is: 'What will happen when I am gone?'

Yet another concept that requires examination is that of 'community'. It is too readily assumed that people in a day or residential unit on a hospital site are not 'in the community', while a unit in a public street is automatically regarded as part of 'the community'. Studies of the use of shops, pubs, swimming baths, bingo halls, or cinemas, and of contacts with relatives or volunteers, may or may not bear this out. Very often, the limiting factor is not the situation of the unit but the impairments of the attenders or inmates. We should be looking towards a network of services, all of which are oriented towards the fullest possible use of facilities available to everyone in the local population. Segregated facilities may occasionally have to be used but they should be prescribed according to individual need, and for the briefest possible period.

Units for the provision of care

Service units can most conveniently be considered under two headings: daytime units, which are concerned principally with occupational problems, and night-time units which are principally set up to provide residential accommodation. This classification immediately indicates how impossible it is to categorize the problems of disabled people but, as we shall see, there is no *necessity* for such categories to be rigid or inflexible if those responsible for providing services remain aware of the ultimate purposes of the whole network of units.

It is clear from Chapter 4 that some hostels provide 'total' care, in the sense that both types of function are provided for on one site. Group homes whose tenants do not go out are in a similar position. Many hospitals, by contrast, because of the size of the site and the multiplicity of buildings, can allow a substantial degree of differentiation of function. The same is true of some large complexes administered by local authorities; particularly for the elderly mental infirm and the mentally retarded. The distinctions between the various types of residential unit are becoming increasingly blurred except in terms of severity of behaviour disturbance or disability or need for basic nursing care, and there is considerable overlap even on these factors.

We shall assume that, in general, daytime and residential units should be separate from each other. In the case of the most severely disturbed or disabled people, it is most convenient for both types of unit to be available on one site, with reasonably large grounds not immediately in the public eye. If they are not on one site, and residents are too disabled or disturbed to use public transport, movement between units presents a serious and expensive problem. Another advantage of a single site is that extra staff are available in emergencies and more flexible staff dispositions are possible. These considerations do not apply when residents and attenders are less disabled or disturbed, although there are problems of supervision and interaction between staff in separate units which we shall discuss in a later section.

Residential settings

The spectrum of residential care is well covered in this book. It includes the hospital ward, hospital–hostel, hostel, nursing home, group home (with more or less supervision), supervised lodgings, flats and bedsitters, and of course the individual's own family. It should be remembered that common lodging-houses, inexpensive boarding-houses, and shelters for the destitute also provide accommodation for the mentally disabled, without always being under supervision or having to meet hospital or social service standards.

The work by Sheila Hewett and Peter Ryan suggests that hostels, in London at any rate, are not developing into old-fashioned 'back wards' as was feared by Apte but that they provide a good standard of accommodation and a reasonably non-restrictive regime. The problem is much more that their aims (perhaps influenced by the optimism engendered by the excellent results that used to be achieved by reversing institutionalism) are still often unrealistically high. As the pressure to accept more disabled people mounts (a pressure which hostels are successfully resisting at the moment), and as high unemployment rates appear more and more to be a long-term feature of industrial societies, it becomes more difficult to 'move residents on'. There is a danger of disillusion among staff as it becomes realized that these high aims are not achievable.

Hewett and Ryan also show that a structured regime in hostels does not retard discharge as Apte thought it might. However, Ryan's data do not suggest that rehabilitation progremmes and the use of 'technical skills' by staff are particularly effective in decreasing disability or increasing independence. This conclusion requires much more investigation and, indeed, the whole concept of rehabilitation is due for reappraisal. Lorna Wing and Judith Gould suggest a more realistic aim of 'management' and the studies summarized by Liz Kuipers point in the same direction.

Another solution, to some extent already being adopted, is for hostels to accept a different kind of resident; younger, with neurotic rather than psychotic symptoms, and perhaps with personality problems as well. It is very doubtful whether this group will respond more favourably to 'rehabilitation' but further work is necessary in order to explore the value of this trend. To the extent that such a change decreases the number of places available for more chronically disabled people who need supervision and support from living-in staff, it is likely to retard the process of opening a wide range of options to long-stay hospital patients.

John Leach has demonstrated the high proportion of severely mentally disabled among destitute men. St. Mungo houses are grubbier than those set up by local authorities and voluntary bodies but the problems posed by residents (many of whom are far more severely handicapped than those in Hewett and Ryan's survey) are being coped with because of the tolerance and experience of workers. More systematic visiting by community psychiatric nurses would, however, have been a great help. Many of the new long-stay mentally handicapped in hospitals and hostels are 'homeless single persons' and in danger of becoming destitute after they leave. We can ill-afford to lose hostel places simply because an ideal of rehabilitation is not being met.

Half the places for destitute men in the UK are provided by the Camberwell Reception Centre. The 'residential' section of this Centre is occupied, in much the same proportion as St. Mungo houses, by mentally disabled men. The intention to close Camberwell, by setting up smaller reception centres elsewhere, is a worthy one but it can hardly be achieved unless much more provision is made, both in the areas from which the destitute men come and locally round the smaller centres, in forms of long-term accommodation.

There are, however, alternatives, such as the long-term hostels supported by the Mental After-Care Association. Many MACA hostels were originally set up in seaside resorts and it will become increasingly difficult to find 'old long-stay' patients who need places in them. There is room for experiment, however, with locally based hostels for permanent residence. Group homes with more extensive and regular visiting by community nurses, with someone nearby on call at night (though not living in), and with a daily home help, would also fill a gap. Disabled people who are living with elderly relatives could be encouraged to use such facilities for occasional weekends or weeks, so that they can be assured that satisfactory arrangements will be made when relatives are no longer able to carry on.

Hostels for the adult mentally retarded, as E. T. Udall and J. A. Corbett point out, also tend to take the less severely disabled. Many might be able to manage just as well in group homes. The experience of Sweden in this respect is worth considering. There are many parallels between the conclusions of Chapters 4 and 7. Udall and Corbett's calculation, that hostels and group homes can accommodate only about half the severely retarded adults in any given district, while the rest are in hospital, raises the question of how much more alternative accommodation should be provided. Hostels and group homes do not take the non-ambulant, multiply handicapped, or seriously disturbed though hostels can cope with lesser degrees of disturbed behaviour. Udall and Corbett quote the story of Joey and his three companions to illustrate the fact that a 'hospital' may itself be a socially rich community, providing amenities and opportunities not easily available in smaller units. The question does not yet have to be decided since the need for more hostels and group homes is nowhere near being met but we shall return to the concept of the sheltered community later.

Local-authority accommodation for the elderly (and, in particular, for the elderly mentally infirm) used to be in large buildings, often former workhouses, and was difficult to distinguish in some cases from equivalent buildings used as hosptials. Even the smaller units now provided in some areas, some of them purpose-built, can take on the atmosphere of hospitals, because the condition of some infirm old people deteriorates, and they require basic nursing care, but it is not possible to transfer them; nor do they wish, having grown used to their home, to move elsewhere. Experiments with supervised group homes are being tried and these will probably provide a useful additional resource.

In the United States much use has been made of 'nursing homes' for the elderly, which are commercially run enterprises with more or less skilled supervision available. Often the fees are paid out of public welfare benefits drawn by the elderly. A substantial proportion of the run-down of beds in US psychiatric hospitals is due to an increased use of such homes. Some of them are excellent; others not so good. There has been an equivalent, though much smaller, use of private hotels and homes for the mentally 'ill' and retarded as well as the elderly infirm, in the UK. We do not think this trend should be encouraged unless a system of licensing can ensure that the standards are as high as those in the NHS or in local authority services.

Boarding-out and family care schemes have been discussed in Chapters 4 and 8. They have not been as popular in the UK as in some other countries, partly perhaps because of a memory of former scandals and partly because they do not seem easy to set up in urban conditions. However, scandals have been associated with every form of residential care for the mentally infirm, ill, and retarded. We now have a fair knowledge of how to prevent the pauperism, neglect, institutionalism, isolation, and cruelty that can characterize poorly supervised and poorly administered services. Such studies of boarding-out schemes as have recently been carried out suggest that, even in urban environments, competent landladies can be found to provide good quality accommodation and care. Further experiments are undoubtedly needed.

In all three major areas of mental disability, the overlap between hospital and other units is clearly crucial. We make some suggestions concerning the organizational and administrative problems in a subsequent section. What needs further discussion here is the concept of the sheltered community. Several such communities have been set up for the mentally retarded and for 'psychotic' children and adults, notably by the Steiner organization, by CARE (Cottage and Rural Enterprises) and by the National Society for Autistic Children, with considerable success.

No one who has visited one of the Steiner communities, with their socially rich environment, their dedicated and enthusiastic staff, and their disabled but active residents, can be in any doubt about the quality of life provided. Somerset Court, the community for former autistic children, is not only a social world in itself, it is also part of local society in a highly realistic and practical sense, because of its market gardening, its use of local facilities, and its support by local residents. Relatives, although often living far from the community, remain in close contact with it and visits home are frequent. However, such communities are expensive, both in terms of money and of motivated staff, and they may be difficult to create in urban conditions.

One possibility is to consider the conversion of sites occupied by hospital or local authority units which are running down. The essential requirement is space for private gardens and walks, with provision for occupation and leisure activities, surrounded by a perimeter of houses of different shapes and sizes, with their front doors opening on to the public street and their back doors on to the sheltered space. Other day and residential units could be situated in the vicinity in order to make use of the amenities. Such a model would be flexible. It would allow many different types of client to be catered for, provide privacy without being remote from community contact, attract (within reason) local people to use its amenities, act as a centre for district services, and foster staff contact and training. Some of the buildings could be leased by social service departments, some by hospital authorities, and some by voluntary bodies and housing associations, although there would have to be a single administration with elected officers and a supervising committee representing all the interests involved, including clients and their relatives. A block of flatlets, which could be used temporarily by people who needed to use the more specialized facilities (rehabilitative or therapeutic) but who required no supervision, could be included.

Ideas of this kind may appear not only novel but utopian, in view of the present separation between medical and social hierarchies, and the proliferation of other groups controlling specialized services. Nevertheless, we think that attempts to overcome professional divisions must surely one day be successful and that it is not too soon to began considering alternative schemes.

Day units

The spectrum of day care facilities is as wide as that of residential units. At one extreme, day hospitals admit patients in the acute phase of a psychiatric disorder who otherwise would have become in-patients. Since it is rarely necessary to treat someone in hospital for more than a few days or weeks, there is also an increasing tendency to transfer to day hospital as soon as the acute phase is over, with appropriate social support at home. Steven Hirsch has shown that this policy can be pursued without greatly increasing the burden on relatives. There can also be a double transfer, to hostel and to day hospital at the same time or sequentially. Plans for psychiatric units in district general hospitals envisage that many in-patients will spend their days in the day hospital, and a separation of daytime and night-time functions is built into the unit. Since most hospitals also have 'industrial therapy' or rehabilitation units, a similar interchange is possible, with in-patients transfering to daily or less regular attendance.

There is a further complication in that people who are frequently admitted to hospital, even though the period of stay is brief on each occasion, often become attached to the ward and the staff and prefer not to be transferred elsewhere. Wards are often used as day units. D. H. Bennett has built up a large clientele of 'ambulant' patients (at St. Francis' Hospital, Camberwell), who make use of ward facilities quite frequently but irregularly, coming in for a meal or a game of table-tennis or to watch television, particularly in 'leisure' hours, as well as on more formal occasions (e.g. to receive injections). Community nurses supervise this attendance, in association with social workers, and thus contact is maintained in a way that would not be possible by using formal out-patient appointments.

A day hospital clientele therefore contains people who are recovering from acute episodes of disorder, others who are socially disabled by neurotic symptoms, and yet others who have more chronic impairments, particularly if there is an unstable or relapsing course. Day centres, and to some extent sheltered workshops and other facilities such as Remploy factories, administered by local authorities, voluntary bodies, or the Department of Employment, tend to accept those with relatively mild and stable impairments but there is clearly a large element of overlap.

Carol Edwards and Jan Carter have made the latest, and to date the most comprehensive, survey of day units for the mentally 'ill' in England and Wales, and they have summarized their findings in Chapter 3. Three-quarters of all the units were provided by area health authorities and one-fifth by social service departments, the rest being run by voluntary bodies. The qualifications of staff, and the staffing ratios, reflected the different intentions of the two main providers but the authors question whether the differences in clientele justify such large discrepancies. The data on the problems of users are not sufficiently systematic or profound to answer the question they raise but it clearly deserves further investigation. As in the case of residential care, the provision of day units has to some extent been influenced by the historical development of separate medical and social services and we shall return to this theme in a subsequent section.

Just as the development of new ideas for catering for housing needs, through the housing departments of local authorities, housing associations, etc., has introduced a different perspective on how the mentally disabled can be helped, so the provision of sheltered working environments could affect day facilities. There are many models to choose from. At Beilen, in Holland, people in family care (i.e. boarded out with families) attend a work centre daily. There is a small, staffed residential unit available on the site for temporary admission if necessary. Many people with stable impairments of moderate severity can work well in Remploy factories or in 'enclaves' in open industry. It may be that some day centres should be upgraded to this level. (Some day centres for the adult mentally retarded have reached a high social and vocational standard.) The work of Donal Early in Bristol has demonstrated what can be achieved by a consortium of interests.

Those living in residential units or at home, and those attending day units, have a need for social and recreational opportunities, particularly during the 'empty' hours in the evenings and at weekends. A number of commentators have expressed concern that many discharged patients are deprived of all active recreational opportunities. Olsen, in his study of the personal and social consequences of discharging long-stay patients, investigated the views of patients, and the persons most responsible for their care, about the loss of the organized leisure activities which had been provided in hospital prior to discharge. The range of activities provided in hospitals and other institutions was not always comprehensive, while the range of interests pursued by discharged patients was sometimes quite broad. The overall conclusion was that all patients—whether in hospitals or other forms of residential care or at home—suffered from lack of social amenities and occupational opportunities. We do not give sufficient attention to the recreational needs of disabled people and assume too low a level of need. Moreover, we rely on traditional prescribed activities provided by services rather than seeking to utilize opportunities which integrate the disabled person into the leisure interests pursued and provided by the community. So far as possible, organizers of 'open' facilities should be educated about the needs of disabled people, and the disabled should be encouraged to use them. However, it must be recognized that many of the handicapped find it difficult to use public facilities and for these special provision must be made. This should include not only traditional social clubs, groups for the pursuit of hobbies and games, bingo, lunch and dinner clubs, the cinema, and outings, but also more imaginative activities in which the disabled person participates actively rather than passively. Examples are the swimming and horse-riding provided for the mentally handicapped, and the sports and Olympics provided for the chairbound. Voluntary organizations are particularly helpful.

The sexual needs of the mentally disabled have received less attention than those of the physically handicapped. Mixed sex wards were introduced into some psychiatric hospitals twenty years ago and a kindly 'blind eye' has often, in practice, been turned on heterosexual contacts between patients and clients using residential accommodation. Nevertheless, few responsible officials are prepared, in public, to advocate the freedom of sexual choice which other citizens now enjoy. Olsen found that a quarter of his group of discharged long-stay patients had a spouse or a man or woman friend and another quarter expressed a wish for such a relationship. Honoré has revived the idea that some form of sexual activity might legally be allowed between severely mentally retarded people and others. We endorse the view that insufficient help is given to handicapped people to enjoy sexual relationships and activities.

Organization of services for the disabled

One of the themes common to all chapters in this book is that many of the functions which used to be carried out on one site, in large mental hospitals, can satisfactorily be performed in smaller units, geographically scattered, but situated within the area they serve. The implications of this common view are not immediately apparent, since we are in the middle of a transition period that may last another generation. The White Paper on services for the mentally ill speaks of a 25-year time horizon. One clear consequence, however, is that the organization and administration of services is bound to become more complicated. Already there is a multiplicity of agencies, each with its own theories and methods.

The ideas behind the organization of the National Health Service, that services should be comprehensive, integrated, and geographically identifiable, should apply also to the network of services—extending far beyond the NHS—required to help the chronically disabled. If this is accepted it must eventually lead to radical changes in organization. In particular, the assumption that medical and social needs can be identified and dealt with separately, which is built in to the present administrative structure, will have to be modified.

It was pointed out in Chapter 8 that the assessment of individual and family need tends to be governed by the organizational framework and by the requirements of agency techniques rather than by the specifics of the presenting problems, which usually cut across administrative boundaries. The emphasis in diagnosis and in care tends to be on the individual patient or client, and family and other important social relationships are considered mainly in order to help explain individual problems rather than as a basis for social action. This means that the importance of increasing ways of coping, and of capitalizing on strengths, both in the individual and in those around him or her, is insufficiently recognized. Immediate relief is the goal rather than relief plus prevention.

The problems involved can be illustrated by discussing the work on residential care described in Chapters 4 and 5. All mentally disabled people living in a defined geographical area should be regularly assessed in order to see whether their current residential setting is the one most appropriate for them. This would include those who have spent as long as six months in hospitals, hostels, group homes, bedsitters, and supervised lodgings. People living with their own families who are severely disabled should also be considered. This means setting up co-ordinating machinery in each area and making sure that there are no gaps in coverage when administrative boundaries are not co-terminous. It means ensuring that people who are not 'ordinarily resident' in the local area are not thereby prevented from obtaining the care they need. A joint committee, including representatives of all the interests involved, is probably the best way to ensure co-ordination and its convenor should be able to collect information both about the candidates for care and the places available. This means, in turn, that each agency should adopt a common review system. When the places available do not match the need, bids should be made to the appropriate authority (often the local Housing Department).

Once an organization of this kind was established co-operation would become easier in other fields of care as well. Common operational policies might begin to be adopted and it might become feasible to consider introducing a degree of joint training for the staff involved, irrespective of their original professional orientation. In this way, whatever the eventual administrative structure adopted a generation from now, the facilities in each area could gradually become organized into a mental health service for the mentally disabled with the aim of raising overall standards towards the level of excellence that exists in isolated units at the moment.

Subject index

advice to relatives 25, 121
alcoholism 8, 93, 96
alienation 94
attitudes of users
  of day units 51 *et seq.*
  of destitute men 100
  of group homes 80
  of hostels 68

boarding out, *see under* Family care

coping by relatives 19 *et seq.*, 33, 112
costs of residential care 82
counselling 24 *et seq.*, 107, 120 *et seq.*, 168

day care 23, 36 *et seq.*, 181
dementia 1, 8, 9, 10, 92, 152 *et seq.*
depressive disorders 11, 41, 114, 116, 155
destitution 14, 61, 90 *et seq.*, 173, 178
disablement 6, 11, 24, 61, 92, 95, 107 *et seq.*

elderly mentally infirm 1, 8, 9, 10, 92, 152 *et seq.*
expressed emotion 19

family care and boarding-out schemes
  for elderly 163, 180
  for mentally 'ill' 83 *et seq.*, 180
  for mentally retarded 106, 180

group homes
  for elderly mentally infirm 164
  for mentally 'ill' 73 *et seq.*, 179
  for mentally retarded 143 *et seq.*, 179
  see also Institutional practices
group meetings of relatives 26 *et seq.*

hostels
  for destitute 95 *et seq.*
  for elderly mentally infirm 164 *et seq.*, 180
  for mentally 'ill' 62 *et seq.*, 179
  for mentally retarded 129, 134 *et seq.*, 179
  see also Institutional practices
housing associations 62

impairments 5, 172–3
  in dementia 157, 173
  in mental retardation 107 *et seq.*,
  in schizophrenia 15, 16
institutional practices 6, 38, 62, 63, 72, 82, 102, 136, 159, 160, 173

medication 2, 22, 104, 123
Mental After-Care Association 61, 71 *et seq.*, 179
mental hospitals
  functions of 11
  history of 1, 2
  see also Institutional practices
mental illness 1, 4, 9, 14 *et seq.*, 36 *et seq.*, 60 *et seq.*, 92, 93, 96, 104, 155 *et seq.*, 172–3
mental retardation 1, 10, 93, 106 *et seq.*
Mind (NAMH) 38

National Schizophrenia Fellowship 24, *et seq.*
National Society for Mentally Handicapped Children 133

occupation
  in day units 46
  in mental retardation 124, 136
  in residential units 70, 72, 183
organization of mental health services 58, 88, 103, 104, 149, 150, 158 *et seq.*, 184 *et seq.*

personality disorders 8, 65, 93, 94, 169
phenothiazines 2, 22, 104
physical disability 8, 9, 92, 119, 144, 153
principles of care 177 *et seq.*

rehabilitation 2, 5, 7, 61, 66, 75, 87, 94, 98, 99, 161, 168, 174 *et seq.*
relatives' problems 16 *et seq.*, 120 *et seq.*
resettlement 2, 66, 97
resocialization 6, 46, 77, 87, 100, 102, 124, 136, 168, 175
restrictive practices 7, 63, 88, 136, 150

St. Mungo Community 97 *et seq.*
schizophrenia 11, 14 *et seq.*, 65, 73, 78, 92, 116, 176
self-help groups 24 *et seq.*, 121

188 *Index*

sheltered communities 180, 181
Simon Community 93, 101
social disadvantage 6, 98, 173
staff skills and duties
  of day units 48 *et seq*.
  of group homes 79
  of hostels 64 *et seq*., 72, 94, 102, 135
    et seq., 141, 166
  landladies 83 *et seq*.

statistics
  of day provision 36
  of hostel, etc., provision 60
  of mental hospital provision 3, 8, 14
  of mental retardation 106, 133
  relating to elderly 152

therapeutic community 2, 94